MUSIC EDUCATION FOR CHILDREN WITH AUTISM

SPECTRUM DISORDER

Music Education for Children with Autism Spectrum Disorder

A RESOURCE FOR TEACHERS

Sheila J. Scott

OXFORD
UNIVERSITY PRESS

Oxford University Press is a department of the University of Oxford. It furthers
the University's objective of excellence in research, scholarship, and education
by publishing worldwide. Oxford is a registered trade mark of Oxford University
Press in the UK and certain other countries.

Published in the United States of America by Oxford University Press
198 Madison Avenue, New York, NY 10016, United States of America.

Library of Congress Cataloging-in-Publication Data
Names: Scott, Sheila J., author.
Title: Music education for children with autism spectrum disorder : a resource for teachers / Sheila J. Scott.
Description: New York : Oxford University Press, [2017] |
Includes bibliographical references and index.
Identifiers: LCCN 2016021613 | ISBN 9780190606343 (pbk. : alk. paper) |
ISBN 9780190606336 (cloth: alk. paper) | ISBN 9780190606374 (oxford scholarship online) |
ISBN 9780190606381 (companion website)
Subjects: LCSH: Music—Instruction and study. | Children with autism spectrum
disorders—Education. | Special education. | Education, Primary.
Classification: LCC MT17 .S4 2017 | DDC 618.92/85882065154—dc23
LC record available at https://lccn.loc.gov/2016021613

9 8 7 6 5 4 3 2 1

Paperback printed by Webcom, Inc., Canada
Hardback printed by Bridgeport National Bindery, Inc., United States of America

To children on the autism spectrum who guide us to observe, to listen, and to teach in new ways.

Contents

List of Figures

List of Tables

Alphabetical List of Songs

Preface

THIS IS A resource book for teachers working with children on the autism spectrum in the approximate age range of 4 to 9. My experiences teaching children with ASD began with a request from a local teacher. She noticed that her students with ASD responded positively to music. She tried to communicate with these students through music but, since she was not a musician or a music teacher, did not feel qualified for this task. Would I develop and deliver a music program for these students? I was excited by this possibility but also naïve. I assumed that all I had to do was consult some published resources, compile their recommendations, and build a program. I soon learned that these resources did not exist.

This publication represents my search for activities with which to create a music program for these children. My educational preparation in both the Kodaly Method and the Orff Approach, my background as an elementary-level music teacher, and my current position teaching courses in general music methods to pre-service educators provided a wealth of experiences to draw on in creating a music program for children with ASD. Over the next several years I worked (and continue to work) with children with autism on a weekly basis, experimenting with a variety of educational strategies, revising approaches, and assessing whether these interventions were successful with these students. All of the materials and activities described in this book were field tested in this program.

My starting point in planning music-based activities for children with ASD was to examine the research literature highlighting the challenges experienced by children with ASD and describing the difficulties they encounter in managing their behaviors in typical school environments. Explanations of these research findings inform the educational strategies described in this book.

Many of the activities in this publication are similar to those already used by teachers. However, this book differs from other resources in that activities are situated in relation to children with ASD. This helps teachers understand how these students learn and, through this understanding, helps students on the autism spectrum reach their full potentials. Readers gain a repertoire of activities to use in their classrooms. They also gain insights into how children on the autism spectrum behave and how teachers may structure educational environments to help these children manage their behaviors. While the educational interventions described in this publication are geared to students in preschool (approximately ages 4 or 5) through grade 3 (approximately ages 8 or 9), the activities in this resource may be adapted for older students.

Many educators work with students with ASD. Some of these students are grouped alongside their typically developing peers in inclusive environments; others receive instruction, or a portion of their instruction, in programs developed exclusively for children with exceptional cognitive, behavioral, and/or psychomotor needs. Many educators are challenged to create educational environments that provide all individuals with educational opportunities best suited to their needs. These teachers may observe that, in general, students on the autism spectrum display an affinity to music. Building on these natural inclinations, educators open doors to social interaction as students engage with others in music-based experiences. Children respond to music in a variety of ways. Their responses involve cognition when children perform the beat and subdivisions of the beat on drums. Their responses involve creativity when students improvise movements to express their aural experiences. Their responses involve communication when children and caregivers interact through performance.

This publication may be used by a variety of educational professionals and for a variety of purposes. Both pre-service and in-service music teachers may use this book to help to prepare music programs for this group of students or to find ways to differentiate music instruction for individuals with ASD. Generalist educators may use this book to find activities that will motivate their students toward joint attention and increased interaction within educational environments and with individuals (teachers, instructional assistants, and peers) within these environments.

The following summary provides an overview of the seven chapters in this book. Chapter 1, Autism and Music Education, provides an overview of autism and advice on structuring educational environments to maximize learning for students on the spectrum. In Chapter 2, Planning for Instruction, teachers gain information about differentiated instruction and creating lesson plans around the principles of Universal Design. Chapter 3, Songs and Singing, begins with a review of research that profiles pitch perception for memory, discrimination, and reproduction in individuals with ASD, followed by a series of practical teaching interventions that assist teachers in engaging students with ASD through songs and singing. In Chapter 4, Listening to Music, music listening is explored as an avenue for promoting receptivity, joint attention, relaxation, and sensory stimulation among children with ASD and their caregivers, concluding with descriptions of educational interventions that motivate students to explore expressive qualities of music such as dynamics and tempo. Chapter 5, Moving, begins with an overview of research literature that profiles the challenges encountered by children with ASD in motor development. This is followed by a summary of the benefits of movement interventions and descriptions of teaching strategies that help children on the autism spectrum practice and refine proficiencies in movement. In Chapter 6, Playing Musical Instruments, the benefits students receive through playing instruments are reviewed including descriptions of the percussion instruments referred to throughout this resource, and explanations of factors to consider when choosing instruments for particular tasks and for particular students. This is followed by guidelines for introducing percussion instruments to students with ASD and descriptions of educational interventions that facilitate the use of percussion instruments with these students. In Chapter 7, Musical Narratives, storytelling and drama are used to integrate the music activities described in earlier chapters (e.g., singing, moving, listening, and playing instruments) into holistic musical experiences. Additional educational interventions are posted on the companion website, along with audio files of the songs notated in the book and an annotated bibliography of picture books based on songs. Updates of research findings, along with suggested implications for education, are also posted. As a whole, this resource provides teachers with comprehensive perspectives for engaging children with ASD in hands-on activities through music.

Working with students with ASD requires that teachers carefully observe and respond to the students' reactions to their educational environments. As I interact with teachers I realize that many of them are challenged to find ways to involve students with ASD in their classes. They want to offer these students the best education possible, but are unsure of how to do so. I hope that the work I share helps educators on their personal journeys, creating and recreating educational contexts for their students.

Acknowledgments

THANK YOU TO Norm Hirschy, acquisitions editor, Oxford University Press, who recognized potential in this work and facilitated its acceptance by Oxford University Press. As well, thank you to Sylvia Dare who so effectively guided the production process. Throughout my years of working with children with ASD and in writing about the activities I use in this teaching context I have been supported and assisted by many people including Jihoon An, Junsuh An, Junwoo An, Helen Armstrong, Bart Brown, Candace Brown, Story Brown, Suki Brown, John Blyth, Sheelagh Chadwick, Amy Jensen, Floyd Jensen, Sunglim Lee, Madeline Lowe, Brent Legg, Mary McMahon, Debbie Schmitz, Ewart Scott, Heather Scott, Joyce Scott, William (Bill) Scott, Debbie Stevens, Jean Valcourt, Shannon Vogel, and Arthur J. Winton. Finally, I express appreciation to Brandon University for supporting the sabbaticals during which I wrote the first draft of this manuscript.

About the Companion Website

WWW.OUP.COM/US/MUSICEDUCATIONFORCHILDRENWITHASD

Readers are invited to explore materials that accompany this book in the companion website. This book is suited to educators with varying backgrounds including, but not limited to, specialist music teachers, special education teachers, and educators in general classroom situations. The website is designed with this in mind by including materials for educators with limited formal education in music as well as for those with extensive backgrounds as music performers and/or music educators. The website includes the following features:

- Updates of the research literature with implications for how students with ASD learn through music
- Aural files of vocal performances of all songs shown in the text in traditional music notation
- Annotated references for picture books that represent songs
- Aural files of rhythm patterns for the movement games described in chapter 5
- Examples of musical narratives to illustrate further the ideas presented in Chapter 7 of this book

References to materials in the Companion Website are highlighted throughout the text using the symbol shown to the right. ▶

MUSIC EDUCATION FOR CHILDREN WITH AUTISM

SPECTRUM DISORDER

1

AUTISM AND MUSIC EDUCATION

The Musical Child

Music is a universal human experience. Children respond positively to music, regardless of whether they possess special talents or aptitudes for music:

> The musical child is therefore the individualized musicality inborn in every child: the term has reference to the universality of human musical sensitivity—the heritage of complex and subtle sensitivity to the ordering and relationship of tonal and rhythmic movement—and to the uniquely personal significance of each child's musical responsiveness.
>
> (Nordoff & Robbins, 2007, p. 3)

Children respond to music in a variety of ways. Their responses involve cognition when children perform the beat and subdivisions of the beat on drums. Their responses involve creativity when students improvise movements to express their aural experiences. Their responses involve communication when children and caregivers interact through performance. The various ways in which children on the autism spectrum interact through music in a classroom situation are described in text box 1.1.

Mrs. Giesbrecht plans music classes so that Marianne, a six-year-old with ASD, is engaged through music in a number of ways. Last week's class began with students singing *Teddy Bear, Teddy Bear* while showing the beat on their laps (see Figure 1.1). ▶

They sang this song, imitating the rhythm of the words while playing rhythm sticks. Later in the class, the students pretended they were bears, moving around the room while listening to Bartok's *Bear Dance* (1931). Mrs. Giesbrecht observed Marianne smile and laugh as she moved around the room, sometimes on her own and sometimes joining hands with one of her peers.

It is widely observed that children on the autism spectrum enjoy interactions with others through and with music (Wan, Demain, Zipse, Norton, & Schlang, 2010). It was originally thought that people with autism who exhibited musical talents possessed unusual gifts. More recent research has noted that, in general, individuals with autism spectrum disorder (ASD) have acute pitch perception (Accordino, Comer, & Heller, 2007). An affinity for music is observed in people on the autism spectrum with sufficient frequency to indicate that the ability to receive and respond to music may be a fundamental characteristic of the disorder (Accordino et al., 2007).

Meaningful relationships with music and making music take time to develop. When children on the autism spectrum are first introduced to music, their interactions may reflect behaviors stereotypical of the disorder: rather than playing a drum in the conventional manner, a child might use it as a vehicle for self-stimulation; rather than moving to express music, a child may rock back and forth to his or her own beat. Through continued experiences, children begin to respond to the musical

Teddy Bear

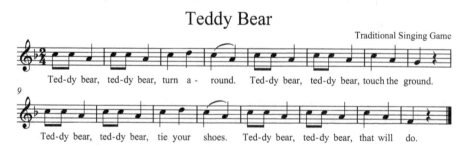

Traditional Singing Game

Ted-dy bear, ted-dy bear, turn a - round. Ted-dy bear, ted-dy bear, touch the ground.

Ted-dy bear, ted-dy bear, tie your   shoes. Ted-dy bear, ted-dy bear, that will   do.

Teddy bear, teddy bear, climb the stairs.
Teddy bear, teddy bear, say your prayers.
Teddy bear, teddy bear, turn out light.
Teddy bear, teddy bear, say goodnight.

FIGURE I.I

TEXT BOX 1.2
CLASSROOM VIGNETTE

Mr. Bennett, a grade 3 teacher, marvels at the progress Jonathan has made. When in kindergarten, Jonathon attended the last five minutes of music class. These experiences were a challenge, with Mr. Bennett gently coaxing Jonathan to sit on his square of carpet while listening to soothing music such as Bartok's (1931) *Evening in the Village* and joining the class in their final goodbye song. After three years of classes in music, Jonathan no longer runs away from Mr. Bennett or tries to leave the room before the end of the class. He participates in 30-minute sessions, playing instruments, singing songs, and playing musical games with his peers.

world around them, communicating with caregivers and showing openness to active involvement with music. Rather than a tool for self-stimulation, drums become objects for interaction as students play the beat in tandem with their teacher and peers; rather than a vehicle for repetitive movements, music becomes an avenue for self-expression. Music becomes a way for students to gain understanding of their place in the world and their relationships with others in their environments. In text box 1.2 we see how, over time, experiences in music influence a student's school experiences.

Children on the autism spectrum display a wide variety of behaviors, cognitive abilities, and social skills. For this reason, no single educational program meets the needs of all individuals in this diverse population. In consultation with physicians and parents, school personnel (administrators, therapists, and teachers) provide flexible supports to meet the needs of each individual. These needs are addressed in a variety of contexts. Many teachers interact with children on the autism spectrum in inclusive settings. In these contexts children with cognitive, psychomotor, and behavioral needs are included in classroom settings where they learn alongside their typically developing peers and, as much as possible, achieve the same goals and outcomes for learning as their peers (Obiakor, Harris, Mutua, Rotatori, & Agozzine, 2012). Children with particularly high needs may be educated in special classes.

Many educators teach children with ASD. Their responsibilities as teachers go beyond the academic growth of their students to embrace extra-musical outcomes such as the students' abilities to manage their own behaviors, to communicate and interact with others, and to gain an awareness of themselves as unique individuals. All children are individuals and no two children on the autism spectrum learn through music in the same way. Regardless of the setting, educators find ways to connect and interact with each child. In this book, strategies and materials to assist teachers working with children in the age range of approximately 4 to 9 are examined. A first step in working with these children is to understand ASD.

What is Autism?

Autism, named after the Greek word for *self*, is a neurodevelopmental disorder (Dimitriadis & Smeijsters, 2011). Children diagnosed with autism display a variety of symptoms and characteristics. Each individual displays these characteristics in unique ways. Some children with ASD function so well that they are difficult to distinguish from their typically developing peers. Other children with ASD are profoundly impacted. Manifestations of ASD are influenced by the child's chronological age and the severity of the condition as well as the nature of interventions and supports provided to the individual: "hence, the term spectrum" (American Psychiatric Association [APA], 2013, p. 53). Autism is more common in males, with only one female in every five individuals diagnosed with this disorder (APA, 2013). Many neurodevelopmental disorders coexist with ASD including intellectual developmental disorders, sensory-integration disorders, and anxiety disorders.

ASD is a lifetime condition with no known cause or cure. Symptoms may be apparent shortly after birth. In this regard, ASD may be the underlying cause for babies who do not form typical attachments with adult caregivers (Dempsey & Forman, 2001). These subtle indications may be overlooked until around the age of two (APA, 2013) when the child fails to develop typical patterns of speech, demonstrates a regression in language skills, and/or displays a marked lack of interest in other people (Dempsey & Forman, 2001). In some cases, caregivers may report that a child displayed signs of typical development through the first one or two years of life (APA, 2013). Individuals diagnosed with ASD experience challenges in communication and socialization that interfere with their ability to perform everyday tasks. Sensory deficits also create challenges for children as they attempt to deal with the sounds, sights, and smells of typical school environments. The classroom vignette illustrated in text box 1.3 describes behaviors often observed in children with ASD.

Throughout this publication, the terms *autism spectrum disorder* (*ASD*) and *autism* are used to describe this condition. This corresponds with the language of the most recent edition of the *Diagnostic and Statistical Manual of Mental Disorders* (DSM-V) (APA, 2013) where a diagnosis of ASD encompasses numerous disorders "previously referred to as early infantile autism, childhood autism, Kanner's autism, high-functioning autism, atypical autism, pervasive developmental disorder not otherwise specified, childhood disintegrative disorder, and Asperger's disorder" (p. 53).

Mrs. Baker is puzzled. Sandra, a girl in her prekindergarten class, does not interact with the other children. When directed toward the music center, her peers excitedly experiment with the sounds produced by musical instruments and spontaneously create their own rhythm band. Sandra plays alone. She finds her three favorite instruments, a shaker, a triangle, and a drum. She lines these up, one behind the other. She moves the instruments into a jagged line and then back to the straight configuration. She would play this game all day if allowed to do so. When Mrs. Baker changes the order of the instruments, Sandra becomes upset, calming down when the correct order is reinstated. Sandra does not seem to know her name but, when asked to do so, can recite the alphabet and the numbers from 1 to 100. Mrs. Burnett consults Sandra's student file and finds that she has been diagnosed with ASD.

The behaviors displayed by individuals on the autism spectrum are defined in the DSM-V according to two categories: qualitative impairments in social interaction, and restrictive patterns of behaviors and/or interests (APA, 2013). Descriptions of behaviors associated with these categories provide educators with an overview of the behaviors they may observe in students with ASD.

QUALITATIVE IMPAIRMENTS IN SOCIAL INTERACTION

Difficulties with social interaction, relevant to both verbal and non-verbal communication, are a defining feature of autism. It is generally recognized that children with autism have greater difficulty recognizing social interactions than their typically developing peers (Centelles, Assaiante, Etchegoyhen, Bouvard, & Schmitz, 2013). Children on the autism spectrum may display a lack of social or emotional reciprocity. They have difficulties communicating their ideas and feelings and they have difficulty understanding the feelings and thoughts of others. These children may prefer aloneness to participation with others in play. They may seek interaction with others as a means to obtain their immediate needs (e. g., requests for food and/or drink) and not for enjoyment through social interaction. Children with ASD may not be attuned to the needs of others and may not notice when another person is upset.

Children on the autism spectrum find it difficult to communicate with others, both verbally and nonverbally (APA, 2013). Children with ASD display a range of proficiencies in their ability to interpret and use language. Individuals more acutely affected by autism may be unable to speak. Students who display a higher level of functioning may be able to speak, but their speech patterns may display numerous distinctive characteristics. Their vocal patterns may not imitate the pitch, rhythm, and stress of their peers. They may speak in a monotone, or their voices may rise in pitch at the end of sentences to reflect the question-like demeanour of spoken English.

Individuals with ASD often reveal a lack of reciprocity in their conversations with others. These children may not respond to topics of conversation presented by others and may abruptly steer conversations toward their particular areas of interest even if these topics are not suitable for a particular context. The way in which a child's obsession with topics of interest limits that child's ability to converse with others is depicted in text box 1.4.

The difficulties individuals with ASD encounter in understanding the implied meaning of language as displayed in humor, metaphor, or irony makes it difficult for them to converse with others. These individuals need to be taught the meanings of the idiomatic speech used by their peers as well as the meanings behind many of their jokes (Hammel & Hourigan, 2013). This knowledge helps children on the spectrum interact with others in social situations.

Body language is a fundamental component of social interactions. In typical nonverbal communication, gestures provide information about a person's emotions and intentions (Centelles, et al., 2013) including the gaze and eye contact commonly used by individuals to indicate a willingness to communicate with others (Innocenti, De Stefani, Bernardi, Campione, & Gentilucci, 2012). Children with ASD have difficulty interacting with others. This difficulty is compounded by challenges in using and interpreting nonverbal behaviors such as observing and interpreting another's facial expressions and gestures as well as a reduced frequency in eye-to-eye gaze. In general, individuals on the autism spectrum use gesture to regulate someone else's actions, to obtain objects, or to engage in activities (Maljaars, Noens, Jansen, Scholte, & van Berckelaer-Onnes, 2011). They make others aware of their wants or

---

TEXT BOX 1.4
CLASSROOM VIGNETTE

Kenny's favorite composer is Mozart. He listens to Mozart's music every day and reads everything he finds about Mozart on the internet. Kenny is motivated by anything Mozart and has memorized many facts about his life and his compositions. Kenny displays many of the behaviors typical of individuals with ASD when in conversations with others. He finds it difficult to look at faces so stares in front of Maria when he talks to her on the playground. Maria excitedly tells Kenny that she scored a goal in the soccer game. Kenny excitedly replies: "Mozart was born in 1756."

TEXT BOX 1.5
CLASSROOM VIGNETTE

Mr. Kwan notices that Holly has difficulty conversing with others. She does not stand face-to-face with her peers, but off to the side. She fixes her gaze downward and to the side of the student she is talking to. The other students seem confused with this unusual body language, resulting in a social distance between Holly and her peers. Mr. Kwan notices that Holly likes the non-pitched percussion instruments and wonders if imitative games with rhythm sticks might provide her with opportunities to practice social skills around body language (see Chapter 6: Playing Musical Instruments). Mr. Kwan holds the rhythm sticks toward his face and in front of his chin, hoping that when Holly looks at the rhythm sticks she will also look at his face. Mr. Kwan wonders if this will help Holly to look at peers when engaged in conversations. He has found no research findings to support this hope but, as with so many aspects of teaching, he uses his professional judgment when experimenting with ways to help Holly interact with others.

needs through the use of simple gestures, such as pulling someone by the hand to lead them toward a desired object or by pointing toward what they need (Paparella, Goods, Freeman, & Kaszri, 2011). These behaviors are on a continuum. At one end are children who do not communicate through gestures and/or facial expressions. Towards the other end of the spectrum are children who interact with others but display non-typical behaviors idiosyncratic of autism such as a lack of integration of verbal communication and gestures. Behaviors commonly exhibited by children with ASD are highlighted by Holly, a student in grade 2 (see text box 1.5).

The difficulties children with ASD experience in nonverbal communication restrict their abilities to communicate with others. Many of these children have difficulty developing relationships with their peers. This lack of interaction takes different forms depending on the age and developmental level of the individual. Young children may have limited interest in other children. Older children (or those more advanced developmentally) may desire peer friendships but have difficulty establishing relationships due to their lack of communication skills and understanding of social interactions (APA, 2013).

RESTRICTIVE AND REPETITIVE BEHAVIORS AND/OR INTERESTS

Restrictive and repetitive behaviors are fundamental features of ASD, impacting the social and emotional development of individuals with this condition (Spiker, Lin, Van Dyke, & Wood, 2012). Restrictive and repetitive patterns of behavior include a variety of mannerisms "such as repetitive language or movements, insistence on the same routines, and circumscribed interests" (Wigham, Rodgers, South, McConachie, & Freeston, 2015, p. 944). These mannerisms are thought to be, in part, linked to the high levels of anxiety generally experienced by individuals with autism (Rodgers, Glod, Connolly, & McConachie, 2012).

Children on the autism spectrum may display "stereotyped or repetitive motor movements" (APA, 2013, p. 50). Characteristic mannerisms include movements in the arms (flapping), hands (clapping), fingers (twisting), or body (rocking or swaying). These children may demonstrate unusual body postures and walk with an unusual gait (APA, 2013). Children may also engage in self-injury such as banging their heads on floors or walls, running towards objects without slowing or stopping, or biting their wrists. The manifestation of rocking, along with a description of how this mannerism might be addressed through music is illustrated in text box 1.6.

Rather than using objects in the manner intended, children on the autism spectrum often adapt objects for use in self-stimulating behaviors (commonly referred to as *stimming*). For example, a child might spin a rhythm stick on its end as though it was a toy top. These children may also be preoccupied with objects and parts of objects. This is apparent when they are more interested in figuring out how to take a tambourine apart than in playing the instrument in the conventional manner.

Children with ASD resist change. They have an inflexible reliance on routines to assist them in organizing their worlds (e.g., they may have a fixed routine when getting ready for school in the morning or for preparing for bed at night). Changes to this routine or to the physical environment lead to extreme distress. This may be due, in part, to their sensitivity to sensory stimulation. Changes to their environment may lead to sensory overload, resulting in situations in which the child is unable to respond appropriately. Routines help children to predict how their day will unfold, thus helping them to control their states of arousal (see text box 1.7).

TEXT BOX 1.6
CLASSROOM VIGNETTE

George displays many of the movements typical of children with ASD. When he enters Mrs. Meyer's classroom, he sits on the carpet and rocks back and forth repeatedly. He seems to be locked in his inner world and does not respond to her when she calls his name. Mrs. Meyer searches for ways to gain his attention. One day she plays a piece of recorded music that is faster than the beat of George's rocking. This music seems to gain his attention. He stops his motions and begins to look toward the source of these sounds. After this first awareness, George slowly begins to take part in the planned activities of the class.

TEXT BOX 1.7
CLASSROOM VIGNETTE

Mrs. Chang's classes are based on the same routines. Every class, children enter the room and sit in assigned places. The class begins with the same welcome song and ends with the same goodbye song. While the specifics of the activities change, the order in which activities occur remains the same. The welcome song is followed by group singing but the specific songs sung change from class to class. Students always play musical instruments, but the choice of instruments varies. The students always look at and listen to books that are based on songs, but the particular books differ. This creates a predictable environment for all students, especially those with ASD.

Going hand-in-hand with an obsession with routines, many children with ASD display an unusually intense focus on specific preferred topics. Children with ASD display a range of behaviors from a preoccupation with specific topics of interest (e.g., brass bands), to non-functional routines (e.g., repeatedly walking around the perimeter of a room), to repetitive motor activities (e.g., repeatedly waving metallic streamers to see how they glitter when moved across a light source). The intensity of fixated interests inhibits the ability to connect socially with people, either through conversation or by engaging in activities that are outside the bounds of these interests.

The majority of individuals on the autism spectrum respond to sensory stimuli differently than their typically developing peers (Baranek, 2002). While the underlying causes of these responses are unknown, unusual sensory reactions observed in children with ASD may "reflect poor sensory integration and/or arousal modulation in the central nervous system" (Baranek, 2002, p. 398). Unusual sensory reactions are an early symptom of ASD; therefore, "these patterns have implications for early diagnosis and intervention" (p. 398). Difficulties with sensory processing may be the underlying cause of many of the restrictive and repetitive behaviors observed in individuals with ASD.

Reactions to sensory input vary from individual to individual and may vary within an individual depending on the situation. Individuals are said to be hypo-reactive when they appear to ignore sensory stimuli in their environment. This description fits children who do not respond to another's voice and/or do not respond when another individual tries to gain their attention by calling their name. Hypo-reactivity to aural stimulus is thought to be a primary indicator of ASD.

Individuals are said to be hyper-reactive when they over-react to sensory experiences. A hyper-reactive individual may be unable to handle bright lights or loud sounds (e.g., music, machines, or conversations). Children with ASD may be sensitive to the sounds of particular musical instruments and hold their ears or try to run away when these instruments are played. Their reactions to tactile stimulation may prove problematic in playing musical games where students hold hands with a partner or clap a partner's hands. Their sensitivity to tastes or smells may create difficulties for these children in the school lunchroom. Problems with sensory perception are revealed in the difficulties experienced by these children when required to coordinate large and small motor movements (e.g., playing non-pitched or pitched percussion instruments), managing their bodies in space (e.g., moving through the open space of a classroom), and managing levels of sensory input (e.g., dealing with the timbres of non-pitched percussion instruments or listening to a variety of instruments when played together). These challenges impact a child's ability to interact with teachers and peers in educational environments. Many children who display repetitive behaviors (such as rocking or hand flapping) are most likely attempting to deal with sensory overload. Such is the case of Michael, who exhibits intense reactions to sounds (see text box 1.8).

Sensory overload occurs when people are unable to separate the details of their environment (the *background*) from the important elements (the *foreground*). Using the familiar metaphor, they are unable to see the forest for the trees (Bernstorf & Welsbacher, 1996). Each detail of an event is equally important to them. They do not know where to focus their attention so they try to attend to everything. Literature highlighting this phenomenon is described in text box 1.9

This over-reactivity may put children in a constant state of stress. They are unable to process incoming sensory information and interpret this bombardment to their senses as threatening (Berger, 2002). Their *flight-or-fight* response prepares to protect them in the face of this danger. They escape into themselves to avoid the outside world. "Often, this behavior is mistaken for 'social avoidance' rather than sensory overload" (Berger, 2002, p. 107). Some children may show aggression or engage

---

TEXT BOX 1.8
CLASSROOM VIGNETTE

Michael is easily distracted by sounds, both inside and outside of his immediate environment. He stops what he is doing to listen to barking dogs or sirens, paying attention to sounds that do not catch the attention of his peers. He screams and runs if he happens to be in a hallway when the school bell rings. In music class he cups his hands over his ears to muffle sounds. The special education teacher suggested that Michael wear ear muff hearing protectors to reduce the sounds in the music room. The music teacher, Mrs. Adam notices a difference in Michael's behavior. He seems more content in the music room when wearing the hearing protectors and is better able to concentrate and interact with her and with his peers.

TEXT BOX 1.9
HIGHLIGHT FROM THE LITERATURE

Kranowitz (2006b), *The Out-of-Sync Child*, may be helpful to readers interested in learning more about sensory processing disorder. Kranowitz (2006a), *The Out-of-Sync Child Has Fun*, provides practical activities to help children develop and refine skills in sensory processing.

in self-injurious behaviors (e.g., banging their heads against walls) when unable to understand and deal with this overload to their senses.

Autism and Education

The mysteries of autism present challenges for educators. Teachers embrace this unknown, seeking to help all children uncover their full potentials as independent learners by shaping educational environments to meet their needs. The development of positive student interactions requires student-centered approaches to learning that motivate these children to join others in making music. Creating a nurturing learning environment for children on the autism spectrum requires deliberate actions on the part of teachers responsible for designing physical environments, educational materials, and interventions, to gain the interest of students on the autism spectrum. In text box 1.10 we see how a teacher's observation of a student on the playground nurtures relationships within the music classroom.

TEXT BOX 1.10
CLASSROOM VIGNETTE

Mrs. Peralta tried many teaching strategies to engage Margarita in music class. Nothing seemed to work. One day, Mrs. Peralta watched Margarita as she sat on a bench beside the school and focused her attention on a bird as it hopped along the grass in search of worms. Mrs. Peralta planned a thematic lesson around the topic of birds. The children sang a song about a bird and moved through free space with bird puppets as props. The highlight was the instrument-playing session, in which Mrs. Peralta introduced the class to a ceramic bird whistle. At last Margarita showed some interest in music class and began to engage in activities with her classmates. This class represented a breakthrough. The bond created between Mrs. Peralta and Margarita remained, helping this teacher to engage this student in other activities focused on additional themes.

While educational approaches may be used to improve the quality of life for children with ASD, no single program or intervention works equally well for all children. Teachers become risk takers, using a diagnosis of ASD as an initial guide in understanding a child's behavioral patterns and then moving beyond the label to see the potentials in all children as individuals. One of the goals of music education is to keep the students engaged as much as possible with music and the processes of making music. The teacher finds ways to motivate each child by providing experiences that are both interesting and challenging, respecting each child's space and using music to guide interpersonal connections. Teachers and students are all learners, joining in musical conversations and, through body language and musical expression, creating positive interactions.

Teachers develop instructional strategies for working with children on the autism spectrum, choosing activities that are challenging but, at the same time, not so difficult that the child is not able to experience success. The resulting learning environment is built on safety and trust so that students are willing to approach new challenges without undue anxiety or withdrawal. The teacher presents music-based activities around guidelines that set boundaries for educational experiences while providing spaces for children to access their own creativity and providing individuals with a sense of accomplishment. Teachers should be sensitive to the needs of each individual, reducing or increasing support in response to the child's actions and reactions as students undertake the tasks that are set before them. As students gain expertise, the teacher helps them to take ownership of their learning.

Students with ASD need opportunities to practice social skills and receive feedback on their progress in order to learn how to interact effectively with others (Gooding, 2009). Experiences in music are well suited to this work because social interactions are integral to much of the music making that occurs in schools. The enjoyment students experience through music often motivates them to continue to participate with others (see text box 1.11).

COMMUNICATION

Regardless of whether individuals are verbal or nonverbal, they have difficulties communicating with others, including difficulties interpreting language and nonverbal information such as facial expressions and gestures. Consequently, even children who are highly verbal may experience difficulties in social situations (Beurkens, 2007).

Music is an ideal medium for providing students on the autism spectrum with interactive opportunities that assist them in building relationships with others (Krikeli, Michailidis, & Klavdianou, 2010; Sausser, 2006; Vaiouli, Grimmet, & Ruich, 2015). Music addresses both verbal and non-verbal forms of expression

TEXT BOX I.II
CLASSROOM VIGNETTE

The students in Mrs. Simpson's music class listen to the piece *Streets Ahead* (Botti, 2001). They move through space pretending they are swimming. Movements emerge from interactions among the participants. Angela and John are always eager to join in. They immediately stand and pretend they are moving like fish. The instructional assistants join them in a movement conversation, copying ideas that are initiated by these children. Julian, who is more reserved, is gently coaxed to participate. An instructional assistant begins by making motions that reflect a swimmer gliding through the water and Julian imitates these motions timidly. His movements become more certain as he continues this interplay. Murray watches what others are doing. An instructional assistant invites him to join in, but he is hesitant to do so. The assistant tries to make eye contact with Murray as she moves to the music. With continued experience, she hopes that Murray will choose to join his peers. As the music ends, everyone returns to their seats and prepares for the next activity.

(Donnell, 2007), arousing the students' interests and motivating them to engage with others in classroom activities (Vaiouli et al., 2015). Through music, students on the autism spectrum gain an awareness of sounds in their environments, the ability to locate sound sources, and the knowledge to identify sounds by name. This includes non-musical sound sources such as sirens or animals and musical sounds such as singing voices and musical instruments. As a means of communication music provides avenues for children to take part in class activities without barriers of language (Nordoff & Robbins, 1971). The shifting combinations of pulse, rhythm, melody, timbres, and expression (e.g., tempo and dynamics) embodied in music provide avenues for nonspeaking communication as social interactions are created through vocalizing, facial expressions, gestures, and movements. Children on the autism spectrum need assistance to become effective communicators through music. Consequently, teachers must be good communicators, able to observe non-verbal behaviors and use this information to guide the learning experiences of the students. Nonverbal communication in the music class is illustrated in text box 1.12 as a means for the student, Vanessa, to choose how she will participate in a music class.

Joint attention

Nonverbal communication often begins with children indicating their wants and/or needs, but not necessarily directing attention toward a particular person (Hammel & Hourigan, 2013). Students may use eye movements to indicate interest. They may

TEXT BOX 1.12
CLASSROOM VIGNETTE

When Mrs. Williamson asks Vanessa which instruments she wants to play, she does not expect a verbal response. Sometimes Mrs. Williamson places two instruments in front of Vanessa and she chooses the one she wants. Sometimes Vanessa mimes playing an instrument to make her request.

physically reach for desired objects. As communication becomes more sophisticated, children engage in *joint attention*. Joint attention occurs when a child notices something in the environment and points to that object, thereby engaging others in what has caught his or her attention. The reward for such action is interaction with a caregiver as they both attend to the object of interest (Jones & Carr, 2004). Joint attention is an early form of social communication that plays a critical role in social and language development. Lack of joint attention is a key characteristic of ASD. Attention to the development of this skill is central to early interventions to engage children on the autistic spectrum with others.

Joint attention is more than a gesture or a gaze. It is a deliberate action to engage another's attention on objects or actions. Joint attention and social development go hand-in-hand. Social motivation underlies joint attention and joint attention indicates a beginning awareness of social understanding (Jones & Carr, 2004). Joint attention depends on building a *value* for social interactions within the child: "In order to communicate intentionally a child must want to communicate, have something to communicate about, have someone to communicate with and realize that communication is enjoyable and can bring about results" (Corke, 2002, p. 10). In this respect, joint attention may be enhanced by building interactions among adults, children, and the children's preferred activities.

One such preferred activity is music. As a non-verbal medium, music facilitates communication without the need for verbal interactions (Donnell, 2007). As children are continually involved in music, they are increasingly able to tolerate the presence of people and may even initiate and maintain interactions. As the children experience the joys of making music they gain satisfaction through successful communication (Corke, 2002). Some students initiate eye contact as they smile and laugh while making music with caregivers and peers. They show interest in musical activities by leaning forward, nodding, and reaching for preferred objects (Corke, 2002).

Play

Children typically engage in several forms of pretend play: symbolic, functional, and sociodramatic. Symbolic play occurs when children use one object as if it were another (e.g., using a block to represent a telephone), give objects attributes they don't possess (a toy bear comes to life), or refer to objects that are not present (e.g., an imaginary tea party with pretend cups) (Terpstra, Higgins, & Pierce, 2002). Functional play refers to activities in which objects are used in ways that are appropriate to their purpose (e.g., the child drinks from an empty cup or rolls a car across the floor while using vocal sounds to represent the engine) (Rutherford, Young, Hepburn, & Rogers, 2007). In socio-dramatic play, a storyline emerges as different episodes of play are put together (e.g., the child pretends to put on pajamas and go to bed).

Difficulties in social communication are likely to contribute to deficits in the pretend play of children on the autism spectrum (Manning & Wainwright, 2010). Typically, children's play is social. Two or more people interact in the spontaneous creation of play routines and games. Through this process, children learn about sharing and taking turns (Corke, 2002). Social play is challenging for children on the autism spectrum who have difficulties interpreting and responding appropriately to social cues. This is why a child with autism may be observed playing near other children or using the same toys as other children, but not engaging in joint interactions (Terpstra, Higgins, & Pierce, 2002). For example, one might observe three children at play in a sandbox. Two children work together to build a sandcastle; a child with ASD sits beside them making tracks in the sand with a stick. This is sometimes called *parallel play* (Terpstra, Higgins, & Pierce).

The social disinterest experienced by children with ASD results in a lack of motivation for social pretend play. This disinterest in pretend play leads to a reduction in opportunities to develop social skills through play. This has broad implications. Positive peer interactions depend, in part, on participation in shared play. Many children with ASD try to interact with other children. However, their awkward and sometimes socially inappropriate attempts to interact may be misunderstood and, subsequently, rejected by typically developing peers. Interaction with others through the media of music (singing, moving, listening, playing instruments) provides numerous ways for students to develop the skills in joint attention necessary for engagement with others in the world of play. In this regard, Kern, Graham, and Aldridge (2006) examined the play of individuals with ASD in outdoor activities. In their study, children interacted with music from two perspectives, a music center and special songs composed for each of the students with ASD and sung by their classroom teachers. These researchers found that, while the students with ASD were attracted to the music instruments, this activity did not increase peer communication. On the other hand, the personal songs helped teachers implement interventions that lead to positive peer interactions. These research findings high-light the importance of teachers in guiding interventions. Teachers provide adult guidance that helps students to learn the roles for play and to practice social skills in a nurturing environment (see text box 1.13).

While the specific ways in which play episodes unfold depend on the personalities involved, Nind (2000) provides a set of guiding principles that describe teacher-student interactions through play:

- Play interactions are enjoyable for both partners. Through joint attention, teacher and students find pleasure through interaction with others.
- Teachers use body language (facial expressions, gaze, posture, movement) and vocal inflections to motivate students and to add meaning to play.
- Teachers respond to what students communicate through their actions, observing and interpreting the messages in the students' nonverbal feedback (facial expressions, gazes, postures, movements) and using this information to guide how the play unfolds. This helps to draw the students into the activities, increasing interest and attention.
- The pace of play depends on the students. Teachers do not rush the process but allow time for pauses and repetitions.

Additional guidelines are derived from Nordoff and Robbins (2007) and Yang, Wolfberg, Wu, and Hwu (2003):

- Teachers are guides, gently motivating the students to take part while allowing them to maintain a sense of independence while involved in play.

TEXT BOX 1.13
CLASSROOM VIGNETTE

Mrs. Wall has two music centers in her classroom. The instrument center contains an assortment of non-pitched percussion instruments; the listening center contains song-books with accompanying compact discs. Children spontaneously form a drum ensemble in the instrument center. Emily sits alone, listening to the compact discs while looking at the pictures in the books. Mrs. Wall realizes that Emily needs assistance in gaining the social skills necessary for play and intercedes with planned musical games (singing, moving, listening, and playing instruments) in which the teacher, along with the other students, provides opportunities for Emily to observe and practice interacting with others through play.

- Teachers build on the students' motivations and abilities to engage in play, adjusting assistance to match or slightly extend the level at which the students are able to initiate and/or engage independently in play with peers.

Music facilitates this process, providing a joint focus for play and a nurturing environment for these interactions. Students on the autism spectrum are able to engage successfully in pretend play when this play is accompanied by visuals such as toys and pictures and when provided with modeling behaviors. Opportunities for engaging in play through music are numerous. The following ideas suggest a range of activities with which students engage through music education:

Singing. In music classes, singing and moving go hand-in-hand. For example, students accompany the song *Rig-A-Jig-Jig* (Figure 1.2) with stepping (2/4 meter) movements and skipping (6/8 meter) movements. ⊙

Moving. Movements provide avenues for students to interact with sounds. For example, students move to the beat of the drum and stop moving when the drum stops (see Chapter 5: Movement and Music).

Playing Instruments. Instrumental sounds portray a story. For example, students play drums to reflect the sounds of a gentle rain or a thunder storm.

Engagement of students on the autism spectrum thrives within a student-centered approach where teachers gently guide students toward playful interactions through music. Students are never forced to be playful. Rather, play emerges over time as a result of positive interactions between students on the autism spectrum and other

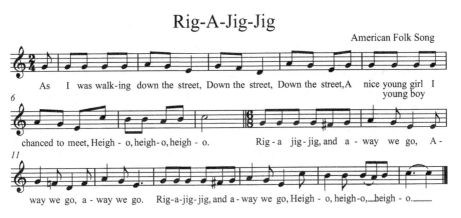

FIGURE 1.2

individuals in their environment. This further illustrates the link between play and joint attention.

Verbal communication

Children on the autism spectrum may have difficulties with verbal communication including the use of words to convey thoughts and the ability to interpret words used by others. They are better able to use and understand language for communicating needs and responding to questions than language used to share emotions and to explain experiences (Beurkens, 2007). In school, children on the autism spectrum are constantly surrounded by talk, including an onslaught of vocabulary and vernacular idioms, coupled with nuances in conversational language such as vocal tone, volume, and inflection. The sensory overload becomes so overwhelming that they escape to their inner worlds. From a teacher's perspective it may look as though the child is not listening but "the reality is that he is desperately trying to comprehend but we are not communicating in a manner that makes sense to him" (Notbohm, 2006, p. 53).

Many children understand spoken language even though they are not able to communicate through speech. Teachers judge the understanding students with ASD bring to verbal communication by observing their use of speech in tandem with non-verbal forms of communication. For example, in music class students step to the beat to show an understanding of beat and its subdivisions. In so doing, they demonstrate their understanding of beat by their actions even if they are unable to describe their understanding through spoken words.

Many students on the autism spectrum demonstrate strengths as visual/spatial learners. As Notbohm (2006) notes, "they think in pictures rather than words" (p. 29). Even young children with ASD respond positively to visual supports. This can take a variety of forms including photographs, drawings, or the signs and symbols of traditional print material. This visual information assists children in a variety of contexts including:

- Describing classroom routines.
- Presenting a schedule for class activities. Pictures show the sequence of educational events such as sing songs, play instruments, listen to music, and line up at door to leave the class.
- Providing students with choices. For example: a child chooses an icon that represents his or her favorite song, picks the instrument he or she wishes to play by choosing the corresponding picture, or demonstrates an understanding of music expression by choosing an icon to indicate fast/slow or loud/quiet (Darrow, 2009).

- Explaining procedures for a given task. For example: Choose a scarf from the box, wave the scarf while listening to the song, put the scarf back in the box, sit in your chair, and listen to directions for the next activity.

Using visual supports children can review and examine the information as they interpret their immediate environment. In contrast, aural information is transient. The teacher provides verbal directions and nothing remains as a reference for the child. Similarly, music exists and is then gone. For example, the students listen to a recorded piece. This aural information moves through time and space until the performance is completed. It often takes children on the autism spectrum more time to interpret aural information than their typically developing peers. When aural information is accompanied by visual representations children have more opportunity to understand, react, and interact with their immediate surroundings in appropriate ways.

Teachers' use of language

Given that children on the autism spectrum have difficulties communicating through spoken language, caregivers simplify the language they use when interacting with these children. Prizant, Schuler, Wetherby, and Rydell (1997) provide the following guidelines for using language with children with ASD.

Rather than relying on language to convey meaning, caregivers communicate as much as possible through facial expressions and gestures. For example, when singing *Row, Row, Row Your Boat* (see Figure 1.3), the leader may ask the students to get out their row boats while making a rowing gesture with her arms. Caregivers may communicate through hands-on learning, using gestures with objects to convey meaning. For example, when asking students to play instruments the leader could hold up a triangle and say "triangle' or, alternatively, hold up the instrument and gesture to the students without providing any verbal directions. In practise, caregivers experiment with the amount of verbal instructions provided to find ways to best help particular students understand the activities in the class. ⊙

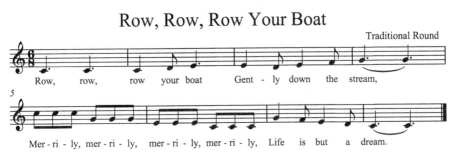

Row, Row, Row Your Boat

Traditional Round

Row, row, row your boat Gent - ly down the stream,

Mer - ri - ly, mer - ri - ly, mer - ri - ly, mer - ri - ly, Life is but a dream.

FIGURE 1.3

Caregivers need to obtain the student's attention before speaking, in part, so that the student is aware that the verbal communication is directed toward him or her. Caregivers might call the student by name. If this does not gain the student's attention, a caregiver might try singing the student's name. The caregiver might be better able to gain the student's attention by sitting next to the student as this action places the adult within the student's field of vision. Alternatively, the caregiver might squat to the student's physical level as this allows the adult a better range of motion to maintain a physical presence in the child's line of vision should the child turn away. Gentle physical direction might be used to gain and maintain eye contact with the child.

Teachers should use concrete language when working with children with ASD. This strategy is well suited to the activities of a music classroom such as:

- What the child is doing: If the child is playing the drum, the caregiver might accompany this activity with language such as "playing the drum."
- What the child is preparing to do: If the child is going to play the drum, the caregiver might introduce this activity with language such as "we will play the drum."
- What the child has just completed: At the end of a drumming activity the caregiver might say "drum is finished."

Teachers may use gesture and demonstration to teach about objects and events in the environment. For example, the teacher might relate the word *lullaby* to the song *All the Pretty Little Horses* (see Figure 1.4) while rocking a baby (represented by a stuffed animal or a doll). Or, the teacher might demonstrate motions used for marching around the room, adding gestures to invite the students to imitate these actions. ▶

Finally, teachers should use the speaking voice to promote a positive learning environment. When working with individuals on the autism spectrum, caregivers use a speaking tone and volume similar to that used in conversations with typically developing individuals. Caregivers may need to speak slowly and in short sentences so that students with ASD are better able to grasp the meaning of spoken language. Emphasis on quiet voices for classroom communication may also positively impact how children on the autism spectrum engage in small-group work with peers.

SCHOOL ENVIRONMENTS

School environments present special challenges for children on the autism spectrum: brightly lit spaces, mazes of hallways, crowds of people moving in various directions, large gymnasiums and/or cafeterias, and classrooms filled with desks,

All the Pretty Little Horses

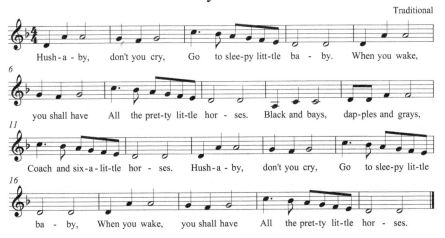

Traditional

Hush-a-by, don't you cry, Go to slee-py litt-tle ba - by. When you wake,
you shall have All the pret-ty lit-tle hor - ses. Black and bays, dap-ples and grays,
Coach and six-a-lit-tle hor - ses. Hush-a-by, don't you cry, Go to slee-py lit-tle
ba - by, When you wake, you shall have All the pret-ty lit-tle hor - ses.

FIGURE 1.4

tables, chairs, and white boards. Children on the autism spectrum may be distracted by the acoustics of school environments (Zhang & Griffin, 2007). Sounds of laughter from children on the playground or sounds in the hallways as children in other classes move from one place to another may make it difficult for children on the autism spectrum to concentrate on the tasks they are expected to complete in their classrooms (Darrow, 2009).

School spaces create sensory overload for students who are unable to separate all the details in the environment from what is important to attend to at the particular moment. For example, if the music classroom has little or no free space, posters on all the walls, and musical symbols hanging from the ceiling the child may be so distracted by this environment as to be unable to focus on the class. This section will examine school environments by looking at ways in which students may be distracted by the complexity of these surroundings and how these environments may be altered to minimize sensory overload. This is followed by a review of how educators might create a sense of belonging within school spaces for children on the autism spectrum.

Sensory challenges

Music is a curricular area in which children respond to four kinds of information: aural, tactile, psychomotor, and visual. Music is in a unique position to present children with a variety of sounds. Singing voices, musical instruments, and recorded music each present possibilities for sensory overload within the school environment. An understanding of over-reactivity helps teachers create a safe learning environment for these students. By observing children's responses to music (e.g., vocalizations, facial expressions, and gestures), teachers learn which students are sensitive to particular stimuli and alter the educational environment in response to these needs. For example, if a child is sensitive to metal instruments, the teacher might use these sounds sparingly; if a child becomes upset when recorded music is played, the teacher might choose short selections for the listening portion of the class. As the children have continued experiences, they might become accustomed to this environment over time; as teachers become more aware of their students' reactions, they can predict and alter the environment to alleviate problems (Hammel & Hourigan, 2011). Teachers also become sensitive to the sensory limits of their students and arrange quiet places where they can unwind. Hammel and Hourigan suggest the use of hall passes so that students may take a break when needed and return to the music room without peers even knowing why they left. Lytle and Todd (2009) suggest that teachers minimize noise in the school environment by reducing the volume of the public address system and closing classroom doors that lead into hallways. The loudness and shrillness of sounds produced by some school bells can disturb a child on the autism spectrum. Teachers need to be aware of a child's reaction to the bell and if this sound results in a hyperactive response, to place the child in an area of the school in which his reactions to the sound are not as intense (Lytle & Todd, 2009).

Sensory overload of aural information is of particular relevance for teachers engaging with students on the autism spectrum with and through music, but the overload of the other sensese is also relevant. When dealing with sensory overload, children on the autism spectrum find it difficult to separate the sounds of music from other aural stimuli in their environment (e.g., the hum of the lights, talking, or rustling papers). Many children on the autism spectrum are distracted by the glare of fluorescent lights (Darrow, 2009), especially when this lighting is paired with flooring that reflects the glare (Zhang & Griffin, 2007). Children may also be distracted by the flicker of these lights and may be bothered by the sounds emanating from this lighting. If the room may be illuminated sufficiently with natural light from windows, this may be an alternative to artificial lighting. The use of natural lighting may create alternate problems. Depending on their height, windows may create a distraction as children are tempted to look outside rather than attend to the activities of the class. The space in which I taught presented this problem as it contained windows that spanned the height of the walls and provided an outside view on three sides. My routine for setting up the class included closing the drapes to minimize visual distractions as students' attention was pulled away from music class and towards the world outside.

Children on the autism spectrum are also challenged by other visual distractions. Crowded shelves reveal a plethora of musical instruments that may interest a child more than a folk dance the rest of the class is engaged in; wall displays may be more appealing than recorder exercises; objects hanging from ceilings reflect the sunlight and move back and forth in the breeze; and computer screens beckon from across the room. These problems are alleviated by reducing or removing the visual distractions: reduce clutter in corners, close doors on shelves or place sheets over open shelves to hide the objects underneath, and turn off computers when not in use. Reduce the amount of stuff in the classroom by disposing of unneeded boxes, furniture, and any other materials that are taking up space (Beurkens, 2007).

The removal of unessential materials may pose difficulties for music teachers whose programs are supported by a variety of materials and equipment. The elimination of clutter may be problematic when classroom spaces are inadequate. A teacher whose music space doubles as the multi-purpose room may have no choice but to endure the stack of chairs in the corner of the room. Nonetheless, he or she can turn off the computer or, if necessary, hide the computer under a neutral-colored sheet. Through careful observation, teachers learn how to adjust the visual environment to meet the needs of the individuals who negotiate the visual challenges of music class. For example, when I began to teach children with ASD I laid all of the visual props (pictures, stuffed animals, and toys) on a table. This made sense from an organizational perspective as these materials were easy to access during the class when needed, but created distractions as students wanted to use these objects for self stimulation and, thus engaged, were not interested in the activities planned for the class. I now organize materials in boxes and produce individual items as needed.

Simplifying the visual environment is a first step in creating a comfortable atmosphere for children on the autism spectrum. A sense of belonging is enhanced when there is a specific seating plan for music. This may require that, for each music class, desks, risers, instruments, and mats are situated in the same place in the room and that all children proceed to their pre-appointed place with names attached to that place if appropriate for the particular group of students. Observing the educational environment from the child's perspective may cue the teacher to distractions that might need to be removed or indicate that a particular child be moved to a different place in the room.

Children on the autism spectrum may be overwhelmed by a music room with open spaces, especially if the school environment is dominated by classrooms in a traditional set up of desks and/or tables and chairs. Teachers may add structure to open spaces by designating specific work areas and posting reminders about the tasks that are completed in the specific spaces and the behaviors expected from students while working in these areas. This approach is suited to music teachers with sufficient classroom space to designate an open area for movement and a place (perhaps with desks or risers) for singing. As noted previously, children on the autism spectrum have difficulty discerning what is important when provided with an assortment of sensory information. Designations of specific areas for specific tasks helps students understand what is important at a specific time and in a particular space (Beurkens, 2007).

Once children become familiar with particular school spaces (e.g., gymnasium, music room, grade 3 classroom) they may panic or have a tantrum if faced with any change in the arrangement of these rooms. Some teachers arrange the physical structure of their classrooms in preparation for the school year, leaving the set-up unchanged throughout the term. This creates a sense of comfort for the students. Within this physical structure, changes in instruction reflect the focus for particular class sessions, such as different picture books, songs, and instruments. In general, students are better able to adjust to these instructional modifications when the overall structure of the learning environment remains consistent.

Routine

Children on the autism spectrum thrive on routine. Routines help students organize and understand their school environments. Many individuals with ASD have high levels of anxiety that interfere with their ability to learn. Consistent routines lessen the stress and increase the student's ability to function independently in school. It takes time for children to gain familiarity with new environments. Some students with ASD settle into a new school routine quickly, some students settle into a routine within a few months and for others the settling process takes the entire school year (Lytle & Todd, 2009). Students with ASD are also sensitive to transitions from one environment to another (Beurkens, 2007). Transitions require that students adapt to different spaces, sometimes with different teachers, and new sets of expectations. Children who have difficulties with transitions appreciate visual reminders and cues that help them transition from one school space to another. Routine in the music class also relates to where a student with ASD sits in the classroom. Hammel and Hourigan (2011) suggest that students with special educational needs be placed in close proximity to the teacher as well as to any materials, such as musical instruments, that the student might use during the class. This reduces the number of transitions the student will need to make throughout the music class.

Teachers begin to establish a routine from the first session of the school year. Students may show signs of stress and/or discomfort if this is their first experience in this classroom and they do not know the routine. Instructional assistants are helpful in this situation. They are familiar with the propensity of individuals and may be able to calm students while the music teacher continues with the class. If a student with ASD is removed before the end of the class this becomes the routine (Iseminger, 2009). Based on previous experience, the next time that student attends music class he or she will expect to be removed from this environment in the same segment of the lesson. On the other hand, if teachers and peers are able to overlook interruptions caused by the child's distress, this individual experiences the entire session and a routine begins to take root. Over time, the student may begin to settle into this routine and show fewer signs of distress.

Referring to children with a variety of special needs, Iseminger (2009) suggests an alternate approach:

> ... instead of jumping into the deep end all at once, try introducing the child to music class for only short periods. Start the short period during the ending routine rather than from the beginning. Remember that predictability is key. If you've established the routine for the last five minutes with a quiet listening time, the autistic child will get used to this closing procedure and will correctly predict it. Introduce the child to the last 5 minutes of music class for several sessions. After several successful 5 minute sessions, the child can come in for the song or activity preceding events until finally the child is in music class for the full period. This slow and steady approach can be very beneficial for children with special needs because it ensures success from the start. (p. 29)

The key is predictability. Students on the autism spectrum need to know what is coming next to prepare for transitions. This reduces the anxiety that so often inhibits their ability to function as independent learners.

Student engagement

Children on the autism spectrum often display repetitive behaviors such as hand flapping, rocking, or repeating words or phrases that seem out of place in the current context. These behaviors do not indicate that the student intends to misbehave. Rather, they demonstrate the student's attempts to find equilibrium.

Students who engage in repetitive behaviors benefit from a variety of sensory experiences throughout their school day. Music provides numerous opportunities for aural, visual, psychomotor, and tactile stimulation. Students see pictures or objects that reflect the content of the music, hear singing voices and instruments, move to music, and feel the textures of the various materials used in class (e.g., percussion instruments or props such as scarves and stuffed animals).

When a student engages in repetitive behaviors, a teacher may try to insert another activity to gain the student's attention. For example, if a student is jumping up and down, the teacher may interrupt this behavior by playing a rhythm on the student's favorite instrument.

Teachers may observe that students on the autism spectrum exhibit unusual, perhaps even inappropriate, behaviors and realize that these misbehaviors are not necessarily directed at them. A student's negative behaviors should not be taken personally. A student may arrive at school in a non-cooperative state due to incidents that occurred at home or on the way to school. Teachers and assistants address this with understanding, allowing the student space to restore calm before the school day begins.

As Hammel and Hourigan (2011) point out, students with special needs may not be aware of behaviors that may seem distracting to adults and typically developing peers. These authors suggest that the music teacher create a special signal or gesture that informs children when their behaviors are inappropriate, noting that individuals who are "less affected by their disabilities" (p. 99) often respond positively to low-key reminders to abide by classroom rules. "This respects the place this student holds within the classroom environment, and allows instruction to continue without time spent redirecting the student during class time" (p. 99). In addition, this strategy nurtures positive interactions between teachers and students.

Motivation is a key factor in educating children on the autism spectrum. These students are more likely to participate in classroom activities with greater interest and for longer periods of time when they are engaged in activities that motivate them both intrinsically (from within) and extrinsically (from outside of oneself). Music teachers are encouraged to observe children on the autism spectrum to discern what activities or objects seem to interest these individuals. Motivations can take many forms: some children may be motivated by a favorite picture book or a favorite song, others may be motivated to participate through the use of classroom instruments. As illustrated in text box 1.14, Mary is motivated through her favorite color.

Teachers often find it challenging to motivate students who would rather not participate in class. Addressing this challenge requires trial and error, starting with what the students are able or willing to do and providing appropriate wait time for responses. Teachers carefully observe what the children do and follow their

---

TEXT BOX 1.14
CLASSROOM VIGNETTE

Mary was not interested in music class until Mrs. Collins learned that Mary loved the color pink. Mary's usual props for music became a pink scarf and a pink streamer. Mrs. Collins tied pink ribbons on the ends of rhythm sticks and around the handles of finger cymbals. *Pink* became the key to interaction as, attracted to her color, she increasingly became an active participant in the class. Soon the activities became more interesting than the color and she began to take part in the class even without pink as the motivator.

TEXT BOX 1.15
CLASSROOM VIGNETTE

Landon resists moving his whole body through open space when engaging in movement activities. He sits in place, moving an arm or a foot to reflect properties in the music. Mr. Schwartz does not push Landon to do more as he knows that these movements are appropriate for what Landon can do at this time. He hopes that Landon will engage more as he gains confidence and facility. This occurs in stages: first, Landon stands to show the beat or rhythm in other parts of his body; second, Landon moves on a square of carpet that provides clear boundaries in which to move, and; third, Landon moves beyond the boundaries of his personal carpet to explore the space in the room.

lead. Depending on the situation, teachers may be able to engage students in a small way and build on slight reactions in a positive manner. Such is the case with Landon who, over time, increases his ability to respond to music through movement (see text box 1.15).

Some students with ASD may avoid music by moving away from the group or running into the hallway. In these cases, students are coaxed to return to the group. This may require time and patience from teachers and other caregivers. Corke (2002) suggests keeping materials within the group so that this area of the classroom is interesting and the area outside of the group is unappealing. If a child chooses to leave the group, the child leaves his or her materials for the activity behind. These materials are focal points for drawing the child back.

Independence

Many students with ASD thrive on routine. They need to know the expectations of their current environment and need prior notice of the activity that follows. Given the high levels of anxiety within which many of these children function, routines and pre-determined procedures help them feel safe and secure. However, in an overly-regimented environment, these children may not have many opportunities to become independent learners.

Independence is built by providing students with opportunities to make choices. Students need structured practice in which they are encouraged to make choices and have the support with which to figure out how to make choices on their own. Providing choices helps children maintain their interest in their educational environments. Provisions for choice making do not need to disrupt the overall daily schedule (e.g., the child chooses to watch a favorite movie rather than do math problems). Rather, opportunities for making choices can be imbedded in daily activities.

Open-ended choices, such as *"What instrument would you like to play?"* may overwhelm students who are not accustomed to making choices. For this reason, choice making begins with two (or, perhaps, three) suggestions from which the child makes a choice: for example, *"Would you like to play a drum or a triangle?"* Visual prompts may assist children in making choices (Adamek & Darrow, 2010). For example, children may choose books by using visuals that represent their titles (e.g., a picture of a train might represent the *Canadian Railroad Trilogy* [Lightfoot & Wallace, 2010]). This activity is adapted to individual levels of ability with more independent children making their choices from among several options and children working on this emerging skill choosing from two or three books.

Disruptive behaviors may be reduced as children become empowered through choice-making opportunities. For example, upon entering the classroom, a student could choose to either sit in a chair or on the floor (Iseminger, 2009). This provides the child with options while, at the same time, allows the teacher to set boundaries for these choices. Similarly, students may be allowed breaks throughout the day to engage in personal interests such as listening to favorite music. Scheduled breaks give children periods of time to lower their anxiety levels. This helps them to be more focused during periods of concentrated work, provided that the time periods for personal interests are clearly delineated and that time limits are enforced. While it is important to be responsive to the needs of each individual, this does not mean that the child has his or her wants met at all times. A common outcome for education is for children to interact in social environments. This will not be achieved if the child is allowed to withdraw from social engagements at will. It is important to coax a child into classroom activities while being sensitive to instances in which the child needs a break from the current environment to regain his or her equilibrium.

DEVELOPING RELATIONSHIPS WITH INSTRUCTIONAL ASSISTANTS

As valued members of students' educational teams, instructional assistants (also referred to as *educational assistants* or *paraprofessionals*) provide support for students with ASD in many areas of development. Instructional assistants help students achieve academic outcomes when they work jointly with educators to shape whole group instruction to meet the needs of particular students. They also help students manage their behaviors and, when appropriate, provide students with personal care (Brock & Carter, 2013). Instructional assistants often help students acquire skills in communication.

There is no single way for instructional assistants to function in school environments. In some schools these workers accompany particular students throughout the school day, including regular classroom environments and out-of-school periods such as bus time (before and after school) and lunch. In many educational environments, these individuals accompany children to music class. Here, they serve as valuable resources, helping music teachers follow through with routines established in other subject areas. This is especially important for children with ASD who have difficulties adjusting to unfamiliar environments. Instructional assistants may also support students with activities (e.g., playing instruments hand-over-hand [for definition see text box 1.16]) and may help music teachers adapt teaching strategies based on the assistant's experiences with students in other contexts.

Katz (2012) structures inclusive classrooms so that all adults in the room support the learning of all students. Instructional assistants are not assigned to particular children, but to classes in which students with special educational needs are members. When all children are involved in peer interactions, both the teacher and the assistant(s) monitor the groups, helping all students to stay on task and supporting the peer interactions of all. If the instructional assistant is helping a group of typically developing students, then the teacher may assist a student with special needs. Conversely, if the teacher is working with typically developing students, the assistant may help a student with special needs. From this perspective, all children are seen as equal members in the school community. This approach reduces the possible stigma associated with those students who need support from an educational assistant.

Maximum student growth depends on successful collaborations among teachers and instructional assistants. Instructional assistants who work one-on-one with particular students in varying contexts have greater familiarity with those students than teachers, especially specialist teachers (such as music teachers) who do not work with these students every day. Thus, instructional assistants are a valuable resource in providing information about a student's academic abilities and behavioral proclivities.

Having been privileged to work with numerous skilled and dedicated instructional assistants for many years, I attribute successful collaborations to respect and trust. I respect the contributions these individuals make to the lives of students on a daily basis and trust them to work toward each child's best interests in music class.

TEXT BOX 1.16
DEFINITION

Hand-over-hand is an instructional technique in which another person holds a child's hand in guiding the child to complete a task. For example, an adult places his or her hands over a child's on a mallet to demonstrate how to play a wood block.

I hope that the instructional assistants respect the expertise that I bring to the classroom and trust me to guide and support their work in music, always putting the needs of students first.

The development of these relationships is founded on communication. To work effectively in school environments paraprofessionals need to know what particular teachers expect from them in specific environments. The ways in which the assistant interacts within these environments depends on the needs of particular students. Some students may be able to function independently in the music class. In this case, the instructional assistant might maintain a physical distance from the student to emphasize this independence while, at the same time, being available if the student requires assistance. Other students may require help to engage in the music-based activities of the class. Some assistants may feel uncomfortable providing this assistance if they view themselves as unmusical. The music teacher can allay concerns by mentoring the instructional assistants' musical skills alongside those of the students. In some cases, the music teacher may request some one-on-one time with an instructional assistant outside of music class to teach specific skills (e.g., playing techniques on non-pitched percussion instruments).

Educators who specialize in teaching music may be able to draw on the experience and expertise of instructional assistants when creating learning experiences for students with ASD. Collaborative efforts often begin with initial conversations in which teachers explain their perspectives on student learning within education in general, and particularly, within music education. This is a time for mutual communication. Teachers share their perspectives of how to support students in music and instructional assistants share how they see their roles in maximizing students' growth through music. It is contingent on teachers to create supportive environments in which these individuals feel comfortable explaining how music education is congruent to other educational environments and suggesting how music classes might be altered to meet the needs of particular students.

Open communication is an on-going initiative. When instructional assistants accompany students to class, it is important that the music teacher welcome them and acknowledge their contributions to the child's growth through music (Bernstorff, 2001). The instructional assistant may have information about a student's successes or challenges on that particular day or week that may impact how the student progresses or behaves in that particular music class. This ongoing communication emphasizes the team-based nature of education wherein teachers and paraprofessionals work together in the best interests of students.

Chapter Summary

Individuals with ASD generally respond positively to music. This bodes well for their inclusion in school music, either in programs developed exclusively for children with exceptionalities or in inclusive classrooms alongside their typically developing peers. Working with children with ASD creates challenges for educators responsible for establishing learning environments that meet their unique needs. A first step in this process is to understand how ASD impacts these individuals. This is accomplished here by providing overviews of two overriding features of ASD: qualitative impairments in social interaction, and restrictive patterns of behaviors and/or interests. Autism is a spectrum disorder. Given the variations within which autism manifests in individuals, teachers approach interactions with these students from child-centered perspectives for learning.

Educators seek to understand children on the autism spectrum to help them reach out to the world of music making that surrounds them. In this chapter ways in which ASD impacts a child's ability to communicate with others were examined. This examination included considerations of how these children engage in joint attention and how they interact with others through play. These considerations were followed by an examination of how children on the autism spectrum experience difficulties in school environments with an emphasis on the sensory challenges encountered by these individuals in typical school settings and how a teacher's reliance on procedures and routines help children deal with these challenges. Issues related to curriculum planning are discussed in Chapter 2: Planning for Instruction.

Discussion Questions

1. What are the the most important features of ASD?
2. How does autism affect how students with ASD function in school environments?
3. How might teachers structure school environments to help students with ASD be successful in school?
4. How does music facilitate communication and joint attention in individuals with ASD?

2

PLANNING FOR INSTRUCTION

QUALITY MUSIC EDUCATION for children on the autism spectrum requires careful planning. Some children with autism spectrum disorder (ASD) are able to achieve many of the same educational outcomes as their typically developing peers. Other students require educational supports and/or individualized programming to reach their potentials. The nature of these educational interventions depends on the needs of individual students and the supports available within their schools. Programming in music education is examined in this chapter, culminating with two lesson templates. The first lesson template, designed around the concepts of Universal Design (CAST, 2011), is intended for teachers who work in inclusive educational settings. The second lesson template is for teachers who work specifically with groups of children (or with individuals) on the autism spectrum. By reading this chapter, teachers will gain information on student programming in music including devising initial and continuing student profiles and planning music-based lessons for students with ASD.

Programming in Music Education

In developing music programs to meet the needs of children on the autism spectrum teachers adapt the educational environment to meet the needs of diverse learners.

This is crucial to the success of music programs in inclusive settings. Adapting instruction requires that teachers make changes to educational environments with respect to what is taught, how it is taught, and how students demonstrate understanding and growth in response to the educational environment. This chapter focuses on programming in music. Hammel and Hourigan (2011) is recommended for readers interested in information about the collaborative processes around school wide programming and, in particular, the development of Individualized Education Programs.

DIFFERENTIATED INSTRUCTION

Differentiated instruction is based on the premise that all students are unique; they learn at different paces and in different ways. Each student enters the classroom with personal interests and prior experiences. Educators acknowledge and respond to the diversity of all children in today's classrooms by using a variety of teaching techniques and strategies to present the same content to students in a number of different ways.

Many students with ASD are able to acquire the same content area knowledge, skills, and understandings as their peers. They may, however, learn in different ways and at different speeds than typically developing individuals. These students often benefit from working toward student-specific outcomes in areas that support their individual needs. For example, many individuals with ASD experience difficulties when communicating with others. These students may be working toward the same content area outcomes as their peers but, in addition, instruction may emphasize student-specific outcomes related to behavioral awareness and social interaction. In inclusive settings, children who are unable to achieve the outcomes of their typically developing peers may need changes to their educational programming in terms of the environment, instruction, or materials for learning to allow them to participate with their classmates.

Educational accommodations are used when teachers believe a child is capable of attaining the same curricular outcomes as his or her peers, but needs assistance to do so (Darrow, 2007). Accommodations do not change the nature of the assignment or the skills that the children develop (Darrow, 2007). Rather, accommodations are supports that help students complete the same task as their peers. Documentation of the child's special needs, the corresponding curricular accommodations, supporting strategies, and individualized instructional materials provides information that helps maintain communication among the various people charged with the student's educational well-being. Accommodations need to be reviewed at regular intervals to ensure their efficacy and to allow instructors to make practical adjustments to student-centered programming as needed. An application of accommodations is illustrated in text box 2.1.

TEXT BOX 2.1
CLASSROOM VIGNETTE

Melody is easily distracted by the activities of those around her. When Mr. Bancroft introduced a ball rolling activity in music, he directed Melody and her partner to play the game at the back of the room with a screen separating them from their peers. When Melody became accustomed to the activity, the screen was removed. She and her partner now work at the back of the class, where a physical distance can be maintained between them and the rest of the class. This is a successful accommodation because it allows Melody the space she needs to concentrate on her work while allowing her to complete the same activity as the other students.

The educational environment is modified for students who are unable to attain the same educational outcomes or attain those outcomes through the development of the same skills as their peers. The purpose of modifications is to alter outcomes to meet the individual needs of these children and, in so doing, provide supports so they may achieve maximum growth given their personal challenges. In music classes, children with modified programs may engage in activities that differ from those of their peers. For example, a nonspeaking child might use scarves to dramatize a vocal performance or maracas to add an instrumental accompaniment while the other students sing.

A first step in developing education programs in music is to gain information about the background of individual students. Teachers may consult individualized education programs if these documents have been developed for particular students. Teachers may gain information about a student's interests and/or proficiencies in music by talking to people who are familiar with that individual (e.g., parents, teachers, or therapists). Information is also obtained by observing the actions of students and by talking to students who are able to express themselves verbally.

The information teachers collect about a particular student assists in planning individualized music programs and in deciding how to approach learning with this student on a daily basis. As well, information collected from when the student initially began to take part in music and as the student proceeds grade-by-grade through a music program provides documentation of a child's progress over time. Questions that aid in the development of student profiles and program profiles for music education are presented in the appendix as forms that teachers may use when assessing their students. These questions address three perspectives:

1. Student profile (initial assessment)
2. Program profile (initial assessment)
3. Program profile (continuing assessment).

Questions included on these forms are listed below along with description of the information elicited.

Student profile (initial assessment)

The questions in the initial student profile form are used to obtain and record information about a particular student with ASD. The chronological age of the student is noted at the beginning of the form as this information assists the teacher in preparing age appropriate activities for this individual.

1. What does this student particularly like?: When working with a student with ASD, it is important to know if this child has any special interests. By appealing to these interests, a teacher might find avenues for joint attention. For example, if a child is interested in dogs, this topic might motivate the child's interest in music. The teacher might begin music classes by singing hello to the student using a dog puppet as a focus; the teacher might work on vocalizations by asking the child to use his or her voice to describe a dog as it jumps up and down; the teacher might close the lesson with the song *How much is that doggie in the window* (Trapani, 2004).

2. What does this student particularly dislike?: Having information about what a student dislikes helps the teacher create a positive environment for this individual. For example, if a student dislikes spiders, the music teacher might avoid the song *The Eency Weency Spider* (see Figure 2.1); if the student is scared of water the teacher might avoid the song *Rain, Rain, Go Away* (see Figure 2.2). ▶ ▶

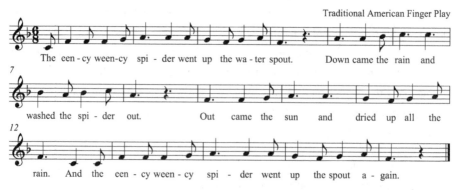

The Eency Weency Spider

Traditional American Finger Play

The een-cy ween-cy spi-der went up the wa-ter spout. Down came the rain and

washed the spi-der out. Out came the sun and dried up all the

rain. And the een-cy ween-cy spi-der went up the spout a-gain.

FIGURE 2.1

Rain, Rain, Go Away

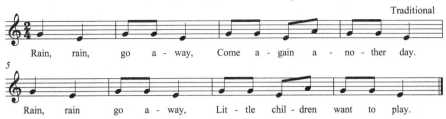

FIGURE 2.2

Whether a teacher avoids a particular topic depends, in part, on the nature of the topic. It makes sense for the teacher to avoid songs about spiders as this topic is not essential to an understanding of music. Other objects or situations that students dislike may be more difficult to avoid when developing well-rounded music experiences. For example, if a student has an aversion to metal-type sounds, an avoidance of instruments that produce metal sounds restricts the non-pitched percussion instruments used in the class and limits choices in recorded music. In this case, the teacher may not be able to avoid these instruments altogether. However, such instruments may be introduced carefully, perhaps by restricting the amount of time spent with these instruments and preparing to move quickly to an alternate activity if the student appears distressed. Short introductions over time may allow the child to adjust to these sounds.

3. In what situations does this student engage in joint attention?: Teachers may be better able to connect with students with ASD if they are aware of situations in which these students engage in joint attention. For example, if a child previously showed joint attention when playing with balls on the playground, then playing with balls may provide an avenue for joint attention in music. If a child seems unable to engage jointly with others, the teacher may look to objects or situations that the student likes as cues for music-based activities that will promote joint attention. If the student is interested in dogs, for instance, then activities such as those described in question 1 might be a starting point for nurturing joint attention with this student.

4. How does this student respond to language?: A teacher plans differently if working with a student who is able to understand and comply with spoken directions than with a student who is unable to do so. In the latter case, the teacher may use visuals (e.g., illustrations, pictures, or photographs) and concrete objects (e.g., props such as stuffed animals) to supplement verbal instructions.

5. How does this student use language?: Information about a student's use of language provides information about how the student might respond to activities in a music classroom. For example, a child with verbal abilities might be urged to participate with group singing. The teacher is aware that a nonverbal student may have difficulties engaging verbally in this activity.

6. Describe any repetitive motions (e.g., rocking, flapping hands) typically demonstrated by this student: Once apprised of the behaviors generally observed from a student in other educational environments, a teacher can judge whether behaviors observed in music class are typical of this student or are, in some way, linked to this class. For example, hand flapping is a behavior commonly observed in individuals with ASD when overwhelmed by situations. If this student only flaps his or her hands when in music class, the music teacher will try to determine why music class initiates this behavior and how the music environment could be changed to ease the student's distress.

7. In what situations, in any, might this student engage in behaviors that may cause injury to the student and/or to others?: If a student demonstrates a tendency toward self-injury or injuring others, it is important that teachers are apprised of these behaviors and the types of situations that precipitate them. With this information, a teacher may be able to intercede before behaviors escalate. For example, suppose a student tends to jump up and down when he or she begins to be overwhelmed. If this state of distress continues, the student runs toward the nearest wall, crashing head first to a sudden stop. A teacher aware of the potential for the initiating behavior to escalate will intervene as soon as the student's actions indicate that he or she is distressed. If the teacher's prior experience with this student is limited, the individual might be removed from the classroom and taken to a quiet area to regain equilibrium. This provides the teacher time to consider possible reasons for this behavior and adjust programming in an attempt to avoid future behavioral problems. If the teacher has had previous experience with this student, the teacher may initiate contingency plans for dealing with the behavior.

8. Which, if any, of the following elements of music does this student respond to? If possible, provide descriptions or explanations for your responses: The teacher indicates whether a student responds to four areas of music: songs and singing, beat and rhythm, tempo, and dynamics by choosing one option of the three provided: "yes," "no," or "do not know." Reasons for responses are provided when available.: This information helps teachers in planning initial experiences in music. For example, if a student focuses intently when

listening to his or her favorite songs, then interactions through songs and singing may be a recommended avenue for engaging this student in music class; if a child seems to show affinity to beat in everyday movements, then this may be a place to emphasize experiences in music.

It is possible that teachers may not be able to obtain information that corresponds to all areas. If this is the case, the teacher notes those areas in which information is available for this initial assessment and completes unknown areas as this information is available.

9. Overall, how does this student's interest in music rate?: The teacher indicates whether the student's interest in music is high, medium, low, none, or unknown. The response to this question does not determine how successful this student may be in music class. Perhaps a student demonstrates a low interest in music because he or she has had limited exposure to music and few opportunities to engage in music making activities. Nonetheless, an indication of a student's previous interest in music helps a teacher gauge how the student may react in music class. For example, a student who demonstrates a high interest in music may display more readiness for a structured music-based class than a student whose interest in music is low.

10. What other information will help the music teacher in interacting with this student or in creating music-based programming for this student?: Question 10 provides space for information that is not accounted for in the previous questions.

Program profile (initial assessment)

The questions in this form are used to assess how music programming might benefit this child. This form could be used by a teacher in reflecting on how to adapt or modify a program for this child. It could also be used by a music consultant in helping a teacher to include a student in an existing program.

The form begins with the chronological age of the student as this information assists the teacher in preparing age appropriate activities for this individual. Next, the context of the program is indicated. This could take many forms. It might be a full inclusion classroom in which a student with ASD attends all classes with typically developing peers; it could be partial inclusion in which the student attends classes with typically developing peers for a portion of the school day; or it might be a classroom designed exclusively for students with special educational needs. The teacher might also have an opportunity to work with the students one-on-one.

1. How might this student benefit from this music program?: Teachers develop relationships with students with ASD by focusing on possibilities for success. A first step is to consider how this student might benefit from participation in a structured music program.

2. What strengths do you possess for working with this student?: Positive relationships begin by focusing on the strengths the teacher possesses for working with this student. Together with question 1, this sets a positive foundation of success for both the student and the teacher.

3. What approaches or activities in your music class have been successful when working with students with ASD?: In this question the teacher notes activities past students with ASD responded to positively and whether, based on the initial student profile, these activities might be appropriate for this student.

4. How do you anticipate adapting/modifying music instruction for this student?: While, in all probability, a teacher is not aware of all ways in which an existing program may be adapted or modified for a student prior to working with that individual, the information collected in the initial student program assessment guides initial interactions. For example, if the student is verbal, perhaps he or she will participate vocally in group singing; if the student responds positively to beat and rhythm, initial participation might involve drums and rhythm sticks; if the student is overwhelmed by diverse sounds, musical instruments may be introduced after the student has gained some familiarity with other music-based activities and is comfortable in the class.

5. What particular challenges do you anticipate when working with this student?: Based on the initial student profile, the teacher considers possible challenges and, as much as possible, creates contingency plans to deal with any concerns that emerge from this assessment. For example, if a student has problems managing behavior in new situations, perhaps inclusion in music may be introduced in brief intervals, beginning with approximately 5 minutes and increasing over time as the student gains familiarity with this environment.

6. What assistance do you need in developing and implementing a music program for this student?: What resources are needed to help this student engage with activities in music and to interact with others in musical ensembles. This could be human resources, such as support from instructional assistants, special education teachers, or music consultants. It could be materials, such as props (e.g., plush toys) or a class set of hand drums. This is illustrated in text box 2.2.

TEXT BOX 2.2
CLASSROOM VIGNETTE

Douglas is a student with ASD who is new to the school. Music-based experiences have potential for building on joint attention, extending Douglas' interests in interacting with others through music. Mr. James has worked with other students with ASD and applies this experience when planning music-based experiences for Douglas. He has found that multi-sensory music experiences, in which a concept of music such as dynamics is experienced from aural, visual, tactile, and psychomotor perspectives, have been especially successful for students with ASD. Mr. James plans to motivate Douglas by building on his interest in motor vehicles with songs such as *Down by the Station* (see Figure 2.3). This song is illustrated by Vetter (2009). ⏵

Mr. James plans to introduce additional modes of travel such as hot air balloons with the book *Up, up, up* (Reed & Oldfield, 2010). Before the school year begins, Mr. James visits a local discount store to purchase toy vehicles that reflect the objects in these books, hoping that this will motivate all students in grade 2. Mr. James thinks it may be difficult for Douglas to maintain his interest for the full duration of music class. He contacts the school administration, requesting a paraprofessional to assist Douglas with hands-on activities and to redirect his attention when he demonstrates off-task behaviors.

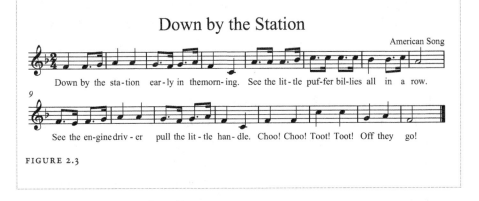

FIGURE 2.3

Program profile (continuing assessment)

This form begins with the entry of the student's age. This reminds the teacher that as the chronological age increases, changes in materials and activities may be required to ensure that the individual engages in activities and with resources that are age appropriate. The context of the program (e.g., inclusion, partial inclusion, other) is indicated, either to confirm the placement formerly designated or to indicate changes that have taken place in the individual's learning environment. For example, perhaps a student began school in a fully inclusive environment, but the placement becomes partially inclusive as the student gets older and is taken out of the class-room for individualized instruction in some areas.

1. How has the student benefited from this music program?: The teacher notes the student's reactions (e.g., facial expressions, gestures, verbal-izations) to music and, from this information, infers how experiences in this class have benefited this student. Students could be asked ques-tions about their experiences either through speaking or other non-verbal means. For example, the student might be shown an assortment of musical instruments and can point to the one he or she enjoys playing the most.

2. From a teacher's perspective, what instructional interventions have been particularly successful?: The teacher describes instructional approaches or activities through which the student has acquired performance expertise and/or gained competence in extra-musical areas. For example, the child demonstrated rhythmic understanding by adapting movements to corre-spond with the changes in rhythms played on a drum or demonstrated joint attention by using rhythm sticks to create instrumental conversations with a care giver.

3. How have you adapted/modified music instruction for this student?: The teacher describes areas in which classroom activities are adapted to meet the student's needs. For example, if a student has difficulty coordinating movements in both hands when playing the cowbell, assistance might be provided by affixing a bell to a stand so the student's only responsibility is to hold a stick and strike the instrument at the appropriate time.

4. What adaptations/modifications are planned for future instruction?: The teacher discusses future plans for adapting music-based activities for this student. For example, based on success with the cow bell, the teacher might plan to adapt the triangle in a similar way. Playing this instrument is expected to help the student refine fine motor movements.

5. What assistance do you need as you continue to develop and implement a music program for this student?: The teacher reflects on the assistance requested during the initial assessment. Perhaps this assistance remains the same; perhaps this assistance is no longer needed; perhaps the student's progress revealed new areas for instructional support.

6. What are your plans for working with this student during the next term (or next school year)?: The self-explanatory nature of this question is addressed in text box 2.3.

Mr. Starzynski has taught school for 25 years. When he attended teachers' college, he was told to *teach to the middle*: that is, to teach toward the readiness levels of *typical* students. Mr. Starzynski found this approach problematic because he was not able to reach all students. Some individuals had already acquired the skills and content knowledge intended to be taught through the activities of the class; other students were not able to engage in the activities designed for the *typical* student. Mr. Starzynski now takes a different approach. He teaches a diverse population, choosing grade level outcomes from the state mandated curriculum and finding ways for all students to take part in learning experiences relevant to these outcomes. He relies on differentiated instruction to personalize educational environments so that all students engage in meaningful educational experiences.

Planning Learning Experiences

In this section, planning lessons that include all students, including those with ASD, begins with an overview of Universal Design for Learning. This is followed by a lesson template that takes into account the principles of Universal Design, and a sample lesson using this template. The chapter concludes with a lesson planning template developed for use with individuals, or small groups of children with ASD.

UNIVERSAL DESIGN FOR LEARNING

The concept of Universal Design emerged from the field of architecture in the 1950s where obstacles to access were eliminated in the physical design of buildings (Mace, Story, & Mueller, 1998). Adapted to education, the concept of Universal Design represents schooling in which the physical, social, and learning spaces include all students and *support all students in meaningful engagement* in the day-to-day activities in their classrooms (see Text box 2.4). Barriers to learning are not thought of as characteristics of the child. Rather than the child adapting to the curriculum, the curriculum adapts to the child. According to Darrow (2010) Universal Design is also known as *Inclusive Design*, or *Design-For-All*. The following is a brief overview of Universal Design. For more information, readers are directed to sources devoted to this topic (CAST, 2011; Causton-Theoharis, Theoharis, & Trezek, 2008; Evans, Williams, King, & Metcalf, 2010; Katz, 2012).

TEXT BOX 2.4
CLASSROOM VIGNETTE

As Douglas is set to enter grade 3, Mr. James reflects on Douglas' progress and notes plans for continued growth. Douglas' interest in interacting with others has grown through the school year. He has learned to play several non-pitched percussion instruments (drums, rhythm sticks, triangles) and enjoys performing music with others. Douglas actively engaged in the *instrumental conversations* activity using rhythm sticks to create interesting rhythmic patterns for his partner to imitate (see Chapter 6: *Playing Instruments*). At the beginning of the school year, Douglas was hesitant to move around the room in free space. Mr. James provided numerous opportunities for class members to move in place, thereby nurturing foundational movement skills for all students, and allowing Douglas to thrive in an inclusive learning environment. Mr. James wants Douglas to become as independent as possible. As a step toward this goal, he arranges for the paraprofessional to attend every second class. He plans to have students work in pairs when there is no paraprofessional present. This is an experimental initiative. If Douglas has difficulty working effectively without the assistance of a paraprofessional, Mr. James will ask that the paraprofessional attend every class. This initiative requires some adaptations to class structure because students will do more work in partners. While this creates an inclusive environment for Douglas, Mr. James anticipates that this will help all students to learn from each other as they engage in hands-on activities in music.

The key to Universal Design is that educational supports are available to all students. This is illustrated in text box 2.5

TEXT BOX 2.5
CLASSROOM VIGNETTE

Students in Mrs. Chadwick's class often work in small groups to create musical compositions. Henry, who is on the autism spectrum, is happiest working on activities in which a clear process is followed to an immediate outcome (e.g., the teacher claps a four-beat pattern and all students play the pattern on their drums). He is overwhelmed by larger projects in which the outcomes are not as clearly defined and achieved immediately. To help students complete this group work, the teacher divides the task into a series of steps with a suggested time frame for each step. The benefits are two-fold: all students have access to learning support (in this case, a step-by-step guide for task completion) and the child with special needs is not singled out as *different* from others in the learning community (Katz, 2012).

Principles of Universal Design

In education, Universal Design emerges from three primary principles:

- Multiple means of representation
- Multiple means of action and expression
- Multiple means of engagement

Each of these components is described below.

Principle I: multiple means of representation

Multiple means of representation is the "what" of learning (CAST, 2011). Through multiple means of representation, students recognize what they already know and link this prior knowledge to their current educational experiences (Evans et al., 2010). This principle acknowledges that individuals differ in the ways they perceive new information. Some students learn efficiently through printed text while others learn better through other visual or auditory means (CAST, 2011); some students are content to sit at a desk for the entire duration of a class, while other students need to move. "In short, there is not one means of representation that will be optimal for all learners" (CAST, 2011, p. 5). This is illustrated in text box 2.6. ⊙

Principle II: multiple means of action and expression

Multiple means of action and expression is the "how" of learning (CAST, 2011). To meet the needs of diverse learners, teachers provide various means for students to demonstrate their understanding and mastery of skills (Evans et al., 2010). This principle acknowledges that students approach tasks designed for learning in different ways and that it is neither necessary nor desirable for all students to express their understanding in the same way. This is illustrated in text box 2.7.

TEXT BOX 2.6
CLASSROOM VIGNETTE

Mr. Hodges considers how to provide students with experiences that represent eighth notes from multiple perspectives. He focuses on aural perception by teaching songs with rhythms that focus on quarter notes and eighth notes (e.g., as illustrated *Star Light, Star Bright* [Figure 2.4]). He visually represents eighth notes with icons *(e.g., stars to represent* this song) and traditional music notation (Choksy, 1999). He models quarter notes as stepping movements and eighth notes as running movements to provide a psychomotor representation of this concept.

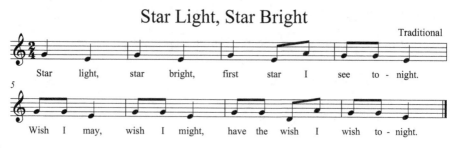

FIGURE 2.4

TEXT BOX 2.7
CLASSROOM VIGNETTE

Students in Mr. Hodges' class express eighth notes in many different ways. They sing songs with eighth-note rhythms to engage aural perception; they read eighth-note patterns from familiar songs presented visually as icons that represent the songs or as traditional music notation; they move through space using running movements to represent eighth notes and stepping movements to represent quarter notes; they play rhythm patterns on non-pitched percussion instruments (e.g., rhythms sticks or wood blocks) for tactile understanding.

Principle III: multiple means for engagement

Multiple means for engagement is the "why" of learning (CAST, 2011). This principle acknowledges that students are motivated to learn in different ways. "The reasons for [these differences] are multiple and include variations in affect including neurology, culture, personal relevance, subjectivity, and background knowledge" (CAST, 2011, p. 5). Some students thrive on routine while others become disengaged in predictable environments; some students respond well in spontaneous and novel situations, while unpredictability creates undue stress for those who rely on prearranged routines to function in school. Some students prefer to work on their own in a quiet setting while others learn best in social situations. This is illustrated in text box 2.8.

Universal Design and Instruction

Guidelines for applying the three guiding principles of Universal Design in instruction are provided by McGuire, Scott, and Shaw (2006):

1. Equitable Use
2. Flexibility in Use

Mr. Hodges observes that some children are motivated when singing; some children are interested in songs when presented as picture books. Some students are excited by playing non-pitched percussion instruments, while the learning of others is supported by listening to and interacting with recorded music. He involves individuals in his classes in a number of activities so, inasmuch as possible, all learners are motivated to take part in the planned activities of music. Sometimes the whole class engages in activities together. Other times they work with partners such as when they create instrumental conversations using drums (see Chapter 6: Playing Instruments).

3. Simple and Intuitive Practice
4. Perceptible Information
5. Tolerance for Error
6. Low Physical Effort
7. Size and Space for Approach and Use
8. Communities of Learning
9. Instructional Climate

These guidelines are presented with a definition from these authors. Practical examples, derived from my own teaching experiences are used to illustrate these practices in music education.

Guideline 1: equitable use

Equitable use refers to educational environments in which all students with diverse abilities have access to meaningful learning in relation to the outcomes of instruction. For example, singing is an avenue for performance in many music classes. Children with autism spectrum disorder may not be able to sing. Nonetheless, they are able to engage in meaningful activities around singing by performing movement activities that accompany songs.

Guideline 2: flexibility in use

Classroom learning accommodates individuals with a wide range of learning styles and background knowledge. Flexibility in use provides choices in how students interact with the materials and with each other. For example, students on the autism spectrum may experience sensory overload when placed within a cacophony of sound. Perhaps these students can complete work in the school's conference room when the class is involved in small group work with non-pitched percussion instruments.

Guideline 3: simple and intuitive

Teachers present new information simply and directly. Music teachers should keep this in mind when teaching young children about meter. For example, rather than providing a technical definition for meter (groupings of accented and unaccented beats), students engage in a variety of activities to help them experience meter. Understanding the verbal definition comes after aural experience.

Guideline 4: perceptible information

Information is presented in varying ways to meet the diverse ways in which individuals learn. Concepts about music may be related to four ways of knowing: aural, visual, psychomotor, and tactile. For example, young students learn about meter. The most obvious way to experience meter may be through the aural sense: we hear music and perceive meter. Meter relates to visual information when the teacher draws a series of hearts on the board to represent pulses, and places accents under pulses at regular distances to indicate the meter (see Choksy, 1999). The meter relates to psychomotor understanding when students explore it through movement. Meter relates to tactile knowledge when children create pictures by placing felt hearts on a board with felt accents underneath to indicate the meter (see Choksy, 1999).

Guideline 5: tolerance for error

Educators know that some students require more time to acquire new knowledge and skills than others. Teachers need to understand that mistakes are a part of the learning process and that some students need more opportunities to practice than their peers in order to acquire new skills. For example, some students with ASD are able to sing the same songs as the other students in the class. However, students who have difficulty speaking may find it difficult to learn these songs at the same pace as their classmates. Teachers may assist these students in acquiring a repertoire of known song material by preparing recordings for them to listen to during free time at school or at home.

Guideline 6: low physical effort

Designs for learning should require that students complete a smaller number of assignments and that these assignments are structured to maximize students' learning. Teachers should think carefully about the skills students develop through experiences in music education. For example, rather than expecting them to complete a large number of examples in which they identify the meter by analyzing excerpts of music notation, students are asked to identify the meter by singing songs while moving to indicate the accented and unaccented beats. Using the latter approach students complete a smaller number of aural examples but gain a more comprehensive understanding of meter.

Guideline 7: size and space for approach and use

The belief that physical space should be accessible to all individuals is fundamental to Universal Design. The following examples provide ideas for how this guideline is relevant in educational settings. Perhaps shelves and cupboards are lowered so that all students have access to materials; perhaps tables suited to the height of typical fifth graders are replaced by tables of differing heights to accommodate the statures and mobility challenges of all students.

Guideline 8: communities of learning

The educational environment emphasizes communication among all members of the learning community. For example, rather than having students sit in rows with all students facing the teacher at the front of the room, it is common for music educators to ask groups of students to sit in a circle on the floor (or in desks). The teacher joins the circle, sitting among the students. This latter formation facilitates communication among members of the learning community. Because students face each other they are able to see what their peers are doing and are better able to direct questions or comments to the group as a whole or to individuals in the learning community

Guideline 9: instructional climate

Teachers and students work together to nurture a positive class climate. All individuals are welcomed to the class and included in the activities of their peers. For example, students with ASD who are unable to speak may be unable to sing. A positive instructional climate ensures that students who are nonverbal are included in class activities. Rather than singing, perhaps these students play musical instruments to accompany the singers.

LESSON PLANNING

Teachers may structure lesson plans in many different ways. They often experiment with different styles and choose the ones that work best for them and their students. Teachers generally guide students' learning in small, successive steps and allow students time to apply new ideas in practice before expecting them to demonstrate independent understanding and before building on this learning with new content.

The same concept may be approached in a variety of modalities (aural, psychomotor, tactile, visual) so that all children have an opportunity to make sense of this content and demonstrate proficiency in ways that best fit with how they learn. For example, the teacher models the beat and children practice their skill in demonstrating the beat in numerous ways:

- Aural: hearing the beat in songs they sing (or in songs sung for them)
- Psychomotor: using their arms to pat the beat on different parts of their bodies, stepping the beat first in place and then through space
- Tactile: playing the beat on a variety of non-pitched percussion instruments
- Visual: seeing the beat through visual representations such as heartbeats or icons that represent specific songs (e.g., bears represent the beat in the song *Teddy Bear*)

Similarly, the same resources provide opportunities for students to learn through these four modalities. For example, non-pitched percussion instruments provide opportunities to:

- distinguish instruments by the sounds (timbres) produced (aural)
- use small motor muscles to hold and to strike instruments (psychomotor)
- identify instruments by the feel of their shape and/or weight (tactile)
- recognize instruments by sight (visual)

The intent is not to reach students only by the modality in which they learn best, but to approach the same content in numerous ways so that students' learning is maximized. By participating in learning through several modalities, students have opportunities to experience growth from various perspectives—aural, psychomotor, tactile, and visual.

The guidelines for Universal Design are not prescriptions for learning; rather, they are perspectives for creating learning environments with full access for all members of the community (CAST, 2011). Teachers apply the principles and guidelines for Universal Design in planning and instruction as appropriate to particular educational contexts. Causton-Theoharis et al. (2008) provide suggestions for curriculum planning that correspond to the principles of Universal Design for learning. Their ideas are adapted here to show the potential for lesson planning that embraces children on the autism spectrum in inclusive educational environments. Readers are encouraged to adapt the format used here to their own backgrounds, experiences, and styles for developing plans and implementing instruction.

Incorporating the perspectives of Universal Design, a lesson is constructed around three main headings:

1. Context (including outcomes for learning and target students)
2. Content differentiation
3. Lesson Outline

Each section is described below.

Context
Outcomes for learning
Outcomes for learning define the larger context for curriculum planning and delivery. The delineation of outcomes for learning involves consideration of what students will gain from specific learning experiences and are often developed or selected in consideration of national, state/provincial, and/or district guidelines. As far as possible, these outcomes should relate to all students' learning.

Target students
Causton-Theoharis et al. (2008) suggest that teachers identify three students who may have special educational needs (denoted as target students) and consider the needs of these students while the lesson is being designed. This ensures that the needs of diverse learners are taken into account at the outset of the planning process.

Content differentiation
Background
Teachers decide what content will be covered in a particular lesson with questions such as:

- How does this lesson fit into a unit as a whole?
- What background knowledge do the students have in relation to the content and skills required to engage in this lesson?
- What new knowledge and/or skills will students acquire as a result of this educational experience?
- How will students demonstrate their understanding?

By considering these questions, teachers acknowledge the diversity of students in their classrooms and seek to eliminate barriers to learning so that all students may achieve their potentials in supportive learning environments.

Outcomes for target students

By devising outcomes for students who have particular challenges (target students) from the beginning, teachers differentiate learning experiences during the planning process. Defining learning for target students is also an effective way to account for non-musical outcomes, such as developing the ability to engage in joint attention.

Content-specific terms

Causton-Theoharis et al. (2008) recommend that teachers provide definitions for subject-area terms used in the lesson. These terms should be expressed in language appropriate to the students' previous experience and background knowledge. Teachers may consider how these terms may be understood through the aural, psychomotor, tactile, or visual senses.

Lesson outline

The lesson illustrated here conforms to the following outline (Manitoba Education, 2003):

1. Activate
2. Acquire
3. Apply
4. Closure
5. Assess
6. Reflect

Activate

During the activation phase, students are motivated by relating what they already know to what they will learn in this session. For example, students are asked to wave their arms over their heads when they hear high sounds produced by a triangle and touch the floor when they hear low sounds produced by a drum. These sounds are labeled as *high* and *low*.

Acquire

In the acquisition phase, students are presented with new knowledge and provided with ways to link this new knowledge to what they already know. For example, through movement students show the contour of melodic phrases the teacher improvises with his or her voice. They relate the motions they made when showing contour to motions they produced when demonstrating high sounds and low sounds.

Apply

In the application phase, students demonstrate their understanding of the new knowledge acquired, and practice skills associated with this knowledge. For example, the teacher writes the first initial of a student's name on the board. The students trace the shapes of these letters with their fingers. They vocalize the contour of these letters using a neutral syllable such as *oo* or *ah* (see Chapter 3: songs and singing).

Closure

In the closure phase of the lesson, students summarize what they have learned. Depending on the questions raised, the closure is an opportunity to emphasize the most important points for learning, clarify misconceptions, and/or provide directions for future learning. The closure also provides students with opportunities to reflect, further consolidating new learning with what they already know.

Assessment

The assessment phase is viewed here from the perspective of assessment for learning. Assessment for learning is the feedback provided to students while they acquire new skills and knowledge within a given unit of instruction. This feedback may take many forms, including the questions raised by students in response to new learning opportunities and the questions posed by teachers to assess the students' understanding of new content. For more information on perspectives for assessment, readers are directed to Earl (2003) and Scott (2012).

Reflect

Subsequent to the teaching and learning process, reflection refers to a teacher's review of learning and/or instruction to make plans for subsequent educational experiences. In terms of Universal Design, reflection may reveal areas in which further work is needed to ensure equal access for all learners.

SAMPLE LESSON: GRADE 2 MUSIC

Context

Outcomes for learning

The lesson begins with a summary of learning outcomes addressed in the lesson. As designated here, letters at the end of the steps indicate which outcome is the focus of instruction (e.g., an A placed after a step in the instructional process indicates that this portion of the learning episode relates to outcome A).[1]

- Students will actively participate with others while making music. (A)
- Students will sing a varied repertoire of music in tune and with expression. (B)

- Students will explore concepts of music through movement. (C)
- Students will read, write, and perform music using iconic and/or symbolic forms of notation. (D)
- Students will analyze their responses to music and making music. (E)

Target students

Three target students exhibit characteristics of ASD.

Grace: Grace rarely speaks. In music class, she communicates by pointing to icons that represent her favorite songs and instruments. She is unable to focus on activities for their duration, often pushing materials away to indicate that she is finished. She works well one-on-one with an educational assistant who gently urges her to complete activities and who guides her back to the group if she runs to the door before class is over.

Jason: Jason's language skills are just beginning to develop. He addresses the teacher by name and identifies preferences with the words "yes" and "no." He is able to vocalize the melody of known song material and has an accurate sense of pitch. He enjoys watching the other children engage in movement activities but rarely chooses to join them without prodding from the adults in the room. Jason needs the security of routine in all school activities and becomes excitable when the usual order of activities is disturbed.

Harvey: Harvey is highly verbal. However, his responses are often out of context as he replies to questions with memorized dialogue from popular films and television programs. He is able to imitate simple pitch patterns. Harvey has a repertoire of favorite songs for which he is able to sing many of the words. His ability to sing the proper melodies for these songs is improving steadily as he gains more experience.

Content differentiation
Outcomes for learning

The letters and numbers stated after the outcomes are used to indicate when lesson activities relate to target students. For example, G1, refers to the first outcome associated with Grace.

GRACE

Verbal: When the music teacher greets her by singing hello, Grace will respond verbally by saying hello or by attempting to imitate the teacher's vocal pattern. (G1)

Social Interaction: Grace will engage with the movement games for the length of time specified for the class. (G2)

JASON

Verbal: Jason will consistently use his repertoire of words. He will experiment vocally by either singing or vocalizing the song repertoire in music. (J1)

Psychomotor: Jason will engage in movement activities, either non-locomotive (sitting in chair) or locomotive (moving in space). (J2)

Self-management: Jason will self-soothe if the regular routine is disturbed. (J3)

HARVEY

Verbal: Harvey will respond in verbally appropriate ways (e.g., he will sing hello to the teacher). (H1)

Verbal: Harvey will sing the songs with his peers. (H2)

Content-specific terms

Beat: Beat is the repeating pulse of the music. In this grade 2 class, beat is compared to steady repeated sounds in the environment (for example: clocks ticking or the tapping of shoes as someone walks across the room).

Meter: Meter is experienced as regular groupings of accented and unaccented beats. The focus for this lesson is an introduction of 2/4 meter as alternating accented and unaccented beats.

Lesson outline

Principles of Universal Design

MULTIPLE MEANS OF REPRESENTATION

- Aural Representation: The teacher sings songs; children learn songs by imitating what the teacher has sung.
- Visual Representation: Accents (<)
- Psychomotor Representation: Students' movements reflect accented and unaccented beats to provide a psychomotor representation of meter.
- Tactile Representation: Children play the drum to demonstrate accented and unaccented beats.

MULTIPLE MEANS OF ACTION AND EXPRESSION

- Students respond to the teacher's singing voice using either voice or kazoo.
- Students perform quarter and eighth notes by using movements in the arms or upper body in place (non-locomotor) or full body in space (locomotor).
- Students perform accented and unaccented beats by moving like animals in response to unaccented and accented beats played by the teacher on a drum.

MULTIPLE MEANS OF ENGAGEMENT

- Improvisational Singing: Students respond to the teacher's singing with puppets, a microphone, or a kazoo.
- Grouping: Individual interactions with the teacher for singing; full group interaction for acquisition and application of new knowledge.

Step-by-step plan

A step-by-step plan to guide teacher-student interactions. This plan includes anticipated responses from children to provide an overview of how this plan might unfold in a classroom. The letters at the end of the steps indicate which outcome is the focus of instruction (e.g., A = first outcome for class; G1 = first outcome for Grace).

ACTIVATE

- Students match the teacher's pitch.
  - The teacher sings hello using hand puppets and plastic microphone as motivators. (B, G1, J1)
  - Children sing known songs (e.g., *Rain, Rain, Go Away*) in place, patting the beat or clapping the rhythm, imitating the teacher's actions to show the beat and the meter. (A, C, G2, J2, H2)
  - Students play the "talking drum game" (e.g., the teacher plays the beat on a hand drum and the students create stepping movements that correspond to the sounds produced; the teacher plays equal subdivisions of the beat on the hand drum and the students create running motions that correspond to the sounds produced, see Chapter 5, pages 157 to 161). (C, E, J2)

ACQUIRE (2/4 METER)

- While students continue to move around the room, the teacher models duple meter (alternating accented and unaccented beats). (C, J2, G2)
  - The teacher asks: "Do you notice anything about how the drum is talking?"
  - Steve answers, "Some sounds are loud and some sounds are quiet."
  - "That's right. The loud beats are accented and the quiet beats are unaccented. Show me that in your movements." Students continue moving around the room.
  - The teacher says: "What animal could we pretend to be through our movements?"
  - "A horse," says Harvey. Students now move as horses. The game continues as children move to the accented and unaccented beats while pretending to be bears and elephants.
- Students form a community circle. Whole Group instruction (based in part on Choksy, 1999). (D)

- The teacher leads students to sing the song *Rain, Rain, Go Away* while clapping the rhythm.
- The teacher leads students to sing the song while using their arms to show the phrases as two rainbows or arcs in the air. They identify two phrases in the song.
- The teacher sings the song again, this time patting his or her knees on the accented beats and patting shoulders on the unaccented beats. Students imitate teacher. The teacher shows the music notation for accented (<) beats.

APPLY

- The teacher claps four-beat patterns of accented and unaccented beats; children imitate teacher's clapping to demonstrate accented and unaccented beats.

CLOSURE

- Students reflect in a whole-group discussion sharing two ideas that they learned today and describing what they would like to spend more time on (E, H1). After this discussion, the psychomotor response to meter is reinforced with the hula hoop game. In pairs, students sit across from each other holding opposite sides of a hula hoop. They sing the song *One, Two, Tie My Shoe* (Figure 2.5) and move the hula hoop from side to side to show the meter of the piece ▶

ASSESS

- The teacher provides positive feedback to help students perform the tasks. For example, the teacher plays the accented beats louder and the unaccented beats quieter, hoping that an increase in the contrast between accented and unaccented beats will help students to discern the contrast in these sounds. She uses verbal feedback to emphasize that individual students are

One, Two, Tie My Shoe

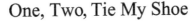

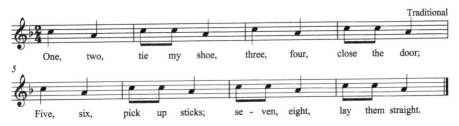

One, two, tie my shoe, three, four, close the door;

Five, six, pick up sticks; se-ven, eight, lay them straight.

FIGURE 2.5

performing tasks accurately with comments such as, "Melinda, you are singing the same melody as me."

REFLECT

- The teacher observes whether students understood the concept of accented and unaccented beats. While most students had no problem clapping patterns of accented and unaccented beats, Grace was off task during this section of the lesson. The teacher decides to review the concept as the motivation for the next lesson before extending the concept of meter to bar lines and measures.

LEARNING SESSIONS FOR GROUPS OF CHILDREN WITH ASD

When I first began working with groups of children with special needs, their classroom teacher suggested 20 minute lessons as this was the estimated maximum time that the children would engage in a new routine with a new teacher and in a new environment. For the most part, the first sessions were comprised of singing songs with accompanying actions. Additional activities were added over time. These experiences guided the development of the lesson template described below.

Teachers strive to keep the students actively involved throughout the sessions. Session length depends on the students' levels of engagement and abilities to focus within this learning environment. I expect that teachers will experiment with the sequence of events to find the order that best suits their students. For example, a teacher may find that a particular child needs extra time to settle into the music session before being able to handle a quiet listening activity. This segment might be placed later in the session to help this student participate as fully as possible.

Lesson planning template

Room set-up

The room is arranged prior to the students' arrival. Blinds are closed so students are not distracted by activities outside this space, lights are lowered, and chairs are in place. Class materials (books, instruments, props) are hidden from view but readily available to the teacher.

Greeting/hello

The teacher sings a greeting to each child; all participants sing their hello song with appropriate actions.

Singing songs

Using icons, children take turns choosing their favorite songs.

Singing book(s)
Children listen to the leader singing songs illustrated in books while they follow the pictures.

Playing instruments
Children play non-pitched percussion instruments in a variety of settings.

Singing book(s)
Depending on the time taken for the previous sections, the leader chooses one or two picture books that illustrate songs.

Moving
Students engage in a movement activity.

Calming activity
Children are involved in an experience with a lower level of activity to help them settle and refocus after the movement activity.

Goodbye
Children and leader sing goodbye; children prepare to leave the room.

Sample lesson
Room set-up
The room is arranged prior to the students' arrival. Blinds are closed so students are not distracted by activities outside this space, lights are lowered, and chairs are in place. Class materials (books, instruments, props) are out of the students' sight but readily available to the teacher.

Greeting/hello
   Materials: Hello song
   Approach: Teacher begins singing the hello song, motioning the children to
      join in the actions and the singing.

Singing songs
   Materials: Icons representing familiar songs
   Approach: Children request songs using the icon board for the selection.
      Movements are added as appropriate.

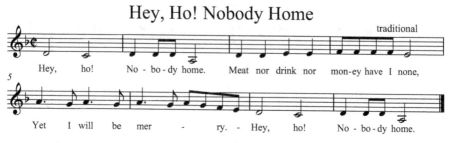

FIGURE 2.6

Playing instruments

Materials: Hand drums (sufficient numbers so each child has a drum; educational assistants may also have drums if sufficient numbers are available); Song: *Hey, Ho! Nobody Home*

Approach: The leader sings the song *Hey, Ho! Nobody Home* (Figure 2.6) and the students play the beat on their drums. ⏵

Singing book

Materials: *If you're happy and you know it* (McQuinn & Fatus, 2009)

Approach: Leader sings the song while students perform the actions.

Moving

Materials: Recording of *Tofu and greens* (Sinclaire, 2003)

Approach: Children dance around the room while playing maracas or plastic shakers.

Calming activity

Materials: *Dance of the blessed spirits* (Gluck, 1762)

Approach: Students listen to the piece and move their upper body to represent birds.

Goodbye

Materials: Goodbye song

Approach: Leader sings the goodbye song while waving to the students.

Chapter Summary

Teachers consider the individual needs of their students when developing programs for instruction. This topic is examined here with emphasis on the needs of children with ASD. Lesson planning is examined with an emphasis on perspectives of Universal Design for learning. The chapter culminates with two sets of suggested templates and sample lessons: the first set is for teachers who work in inclusive educational settings; the second set is for teachers who work specifically with groups of children (or individuals) with ASD. Materials and activities for reaching children on the autism spectrum are provided in subsequent chapters. While all groups of children differ depending on the personalities of the individuals, this lesson template represents the order of activities that was appropriate for my students. Readers are encouraged to adapt this lesson format to suit their own teaching contexts.

Questions for Discussion

1. How do the concepts of Universal Design contribute to planning and instruction in education?
2. How does addressing the same content from multiple perspectives (aural, psychomotor, tactile, visual) help students learn?
3. Describe how particular content in music (e.g., melodic contour, beat, meter) may be approached through a number of modalities (aural, psychomotor, tactile, visual).
4. How might you adapt the style and structure of your lesson plans to address the needs of your students with ASD?

Note

1. Thank you to Dr. Bob de Frece, professor emeritus, University of Alberta, for suggesting this strategy for indicating how curricular outcomes correspond with teaching strategies.

3

SONGS AND SINGING

CHILDREN ON THE autism spectrum consistently demonstrate an affinity for music (Armstrong, 1999). Songs and singing are central to this positive response to music. Children enjoy listening to their favorite songs and are often seen laughing, clapping, and adding movements to accompany the actions of these songs. Children with limited verbal skills have been known to acquire the ability to sing by engaging in continued experiences with songs. Thus, songs and singing have the potential to bridge verbal communication through music.

Many teachers of children with autism spectrum disorder (ASD) know and understand the benefits of songs and singing for their students. To advocate effectively for these students, teachers support their observations of classroom experiences with documentation that explores and clarifies how children with autism respond and learn through experiences in songs and singing. This chapter includes an overview of selected research findings that profile pitch perception for memory, discrimination, and reproduction observed in individuals with ASD. Using these research findings as guides, teaching strategies and selected resources for including songs and singing in education for children on the autism spectrum is described. Suggested songs for use in primary classrooms are referenced throughout this chapter.

Cognitive Perceptions

PITCH PERCEPTION

Pitch perception refers to the relative highness or lowness of sounds based on their frequencies (the number of cycles or vibrations per second created by the sound waves generated from the source). Thaut (1987) noted that children with ASD spend more time listening to music than children without autism. This natural affinity for music may be due, in part, to their enhanced abilities to remember and discriminate pitches and their acute memory for melodies. Heaton, Hermelin, and Pring (1998) found that children with ASD who did not have musical training were better able to identify and remember isolated pitches than children without autism who formed the control group in their study. Heaton (2003) found that children with ASD were better able to remember isolated pitches and to use long-term memory to discern these tones within musical chords than their typically developing counterparts. Heaton (2005) extended this research, finding that children with ASD performed significantly better than children without ASD when asked to discriminate pitch direction (by indicating whether pitches sound progressively higher or lower) in intervals of 1 to 4 semitones.

These research findings have important implications for education. Since children on the autism spectrum have a natural affinity for pitch perception and are naturally attentive to music, it would seem that music is a natural fit for teaching these children both about music and through music. In this sense, their natural attention to music may become a building block to learning. With continued interactions through music, children gain a repertoire of known songs. Through this familiarity many children gradually become more involved in the music experience by performing the actions that accompany songs or singing the lyrics. With instructional guidance they may transfer their understanding of music into other contexts. For example, through songs children can acquire understanding about the concepts of dynamics by always singing some sound loudly (*Bingo* [Figure 3.1]) and some songs quietly (*Simple Gifts* [Figure 3.2]). ⏵ ⏵

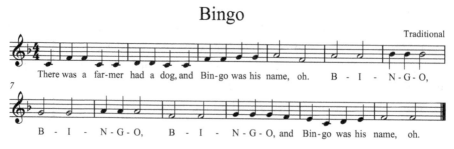

Bingo

Traditional

There was a far-mer had a dog, and Bin-go was his name, oh.   B - I - N-G-O,

B - I - N-G-O,   B - I - N - G-O, and Bin-go was his name, oh.

FIGURE 3.1

Simple Gifts

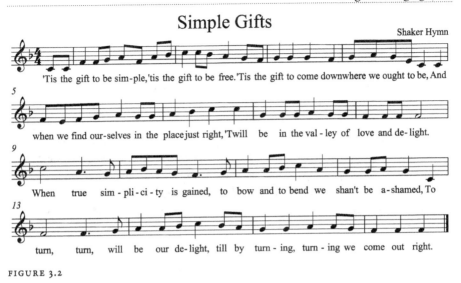

Shaker Hymn

'Tis the gift to be sim-ple, 'tis the gift to be free. 'Tis the gift to come down where we ought to be, And

when we find our-selves in the place just right, 'Twill be in the val - ley of love and de- light.

When true sim - pli - ci - ty is gained, to bow and to bend we shan't be a-shamed, To

turn, turn, will be our de- light, till by turn - ing, turn - ing we come out right.

FIGURE 3.2

With guidance, these children may be able to apply this concept to other circumstances, for instance, by talking quietly in the school library or resource center and talking loudly in the gymnasium or on the playground.

Children on the autism spectrum are not only able to perceive pitches and pitch direction; they are able to reproduce melodic patterns (Lim, 2012). For example, Applebaum, Egel, Kroegel, and Imhof (1979) found that children on the autism spectrum were able to reproduce one to four tones presented in an atonal sequence as well as or better than children with a formal education in music. This research finding is borne out in classroom settings. For example, teachers of music often find that children on the autism spectrum are readily able to use their voices to match their teacher's vocal pitches. Vocal behaviors typically observed by music teachers are described in the vignette portrayed in text box 3.1. ▶

A child's initial vocal responses may be involuntary. With consistent exposure to music, these vocal inflections become "intentional and self-expressive" (Nordoff & Robbins, 2007, p. 227). Vocal responses become a way for children to communicate enjoyment of musical experiences. Students are encouraged to engage in group singing even though their vocalizations may be atypical. Over time, children may begin to reproduce the melody and even the words of their favorite songs. For that reason, these vocalizations are not discouraged as interruptions to the songs, but are encouraged to promote children's active engagement in musical experiences. As shown in text box 3.2, these natural predispositions toward music may help these students develop skills in in-tune singing so that, over time, they acquire a repertoire of songs.

Mr. Jensen, who uses a variety of musical games to help students in kindergarten practice and refine their abilities to perceive and remember music, was amazed by how well Carl, a seven-year-old with ASD, performed these tasks. This student correctly indicated whether individual sounds were high or low and whether successive pitches were moving higher or lower. Even though Carl had limited verbal abilities, he vocalized the melodies of songs using random syllables such as *oo* or *ah*. One day Mr. Jensen was on recess duty. Carl was playing in the sand box, moving a toy truck along some makeshift roads while humming the *Goodbye Song* (see Figure 3.3) using the same pitches Mr. Jensen had used when teaching the song to the class.

Goodbye Song

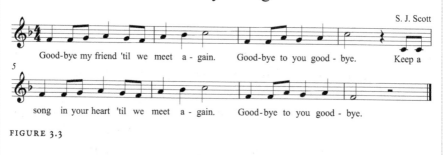

S. J. Scott

Good-bye my friend 'til we meet a - gain. Good-bye to you good - bye. Keep a

song in your heart 'til we meet a - gain. Good-bye to you good - bye.

FIGURE 3.3

The children in Mrs. Russell's grade 2 class enjoy picture books. One of their favorites is *Pete the cat: The wheels on the bus* (Dean, 2013). The students enjoy singing the song and adding words or sounds to enhance the activities portrayed in the story. At first Melissa, a young girl with ASD, did not take part in these vocalizations. Gradually, she began to contribute personal improvisations to the melody sung by the others. Over time, her renditions increasingly resembled those of the class. She even sang some of the words. By the end of the year Melissa joined her class when they sang this song at a festival to celebrate the end of the school year.

RELATIONSHIPS BETWEEN LANGUAGE AND MUSIC

One of the distinguishing features of ASD centers on differences in verbal communication. Approximately one-third to one-half of individuals with ASD do not develop functional speech (Preston & Carter, 2009). These are the individuals who do not communicate through language or who use single words to make requests and to respond to questions from caregivers. Toward the other end of the spectrum are individuals whose speech displays abnormalities such as vocal patterns that do not imitate the pitch and rhythm of typical speakers or whose use of language does not fit the context of a conversation. Regardless of an individual's development in relation to the spectrum, all children with autism are at risk for lifelong challenges in both understanding and using language (Watson, Roberts, Baranek, Mandulak, & Dalton, 2012). Children receive educational interventions with regard to language acquisition as early as possible as language proficiency impacts the extent to which these children integrate into mainstream society as adults (Szatmari, Bryson, Boyle, Streiner, & Duku, 2003). Lim (2012) may be of interest to readers interested in exploring relationships between language and music in more detail.

Research findings guide and support the use of songs and singing to assist children on the autism spectrum to acquire language. Schon et al. (2008) maintain that songs and singing contribute to language acquisition, pointing to the potential of songs to increase a child's "level of arousal and attention" (p. 976). In a similar vein, Shore (2003) shares the experience of working with a child on the autism spectrum for whom all communications were sung. Shore observed that if she reverted to conversation, the child lost focus and drifted into his inner world. In Shore's words "the music helps to organize verbal communication skills that already exist" (p. 104). Related to this idea, Simpson, Keen, and Lamb (2013) found that music created a more engaging context for children with ASD. Children on the autism spectrum show their enjoyment of songs, for example, laughing, clapping, and even joining the group in singing their favorite songs. For some children music is a natural medium for verbal acquisition.

McMillan and Saffran (2004) highlight similarities between music and language, explaining that both are structures that unfold over time and that both speech and language are perceived as patterns of pitches that create meaning through sounds when grouped together. The concept of memory for tonal sequences extends to memory for patterns in rhythm and metric organization (Thaut, 2008). In music, melodic patterns are organized temporally through beat and rhythm and metrically through the use of accented and unaccented beats to organize beats into predictable patterns. Similarly, the perception of rhythm and meter plays a role in speech, such as the placement of accents on syllables and using silence (in music described as *rests*) to separate sentences or make places for commas in speech. Thus, both memory for music and language depend on the ability to recognize and group information into categories or units.

An understanding of the relationships between language in music and language in speech helps to explain why some children are able to respond to language in

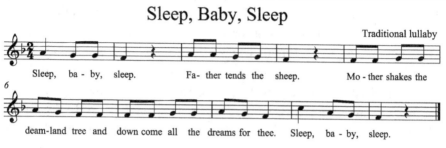

FIGURE 3.4

song more readily than speech. Taking the song *Sleep, Baby, Sleep* as an example (see Figure 3.4), we see a simple structure in the melody with all tones within the range of a fifth, from F up to C. While the words differ, the motive of the first measure is repeated in the third, with a change of rhythm in the melody to account for the words. The third motive, "Mother shakes the dreamland tree," is repeated with the words "down come all the dreams for thee." The first motive repeats in the final two measures, beginning with a higher tone to signal the end of the song. The melody then comes to rest on the tonic. The repetition of these melodic motives helps students remember the song. The melody, meter, and rhythm are predictable. In contrast to speech, where spoken patterns vary with individuals, the song remains constant across time and when performed by different individuals. A suitable tempo for the song may be slower than typical speech, providing students on the autism spectrum time to process this aural information. ⏵

In summary, research has shown that children on the autism spectrum respond positively through music, both in their perception of melody and their ability to respond vocally to what they hear. On a practical level, these findings have implications for education:

1. By paying attention to personal interests, developmental levels, and unique learning styles, musical experiences can be created to motivate children to learn.
2. Knowledge of and interaction with music can influence a child's ability to use language in singing and in speech.
3. By analyzing each child's vocal responses, a teacher can learn what that child is able to do and see possibilities for growth through music.
4. The improvisatory nature of music provides openings for children to explore their vocal capabilities in settings where there is room for personal expression and all appropriate responses are celebrated.

Vocal (Singing) Experiences for Children on the Autism Spectrum

Elementary level general music is founded, in large part, on songs and singing. In many programs, the voice is the child's first musical instrument. While some children enter school able to sing in tune, the acquisition of this skill is an important component of music instruction, with children obtaining a large repertoire of songs by imitating their teachers' vocal models. Teaching typically developing children how to sing differs from teaching children on the autism spectrum, especially when the child's verbal skills are limited. Nonetheless, children on the autism spectrum benefit in several ways from membership in ensemble singing:

- Interacting with adult caregivers and peers in social situations
- Gaining knowledge and understanding of culture through songs and dances
- Having opportunities to explore and manipulate their voices
- Having opportunities to move in response to modulations in pitch and contour in songs
- Having opportunities to move in response to the words of songs

The ideal singing voice for children is "a *light, natural treble*" (Montgomery, 2002, p. 26, emphasis in original). This was traditionally called the *head voice* but in more recent literature is referred to as the *light voice* (Trollinger, 2007). This vocal quality may not be familiar to children in North American culture who are accustomed to hearing a heavier quality of vocal production used by the majority of singers they hear in popular culture (e.g., on recordings transmitted over the radio, television, or Internet). A brief overview of singing in elementary schools is provided here. Readers interested in a detailed overview of research that examines children's singing development and implications for teaching singers may wish to consult Hedden (2012) and Trollinger (2007).

According to Trollinger (2007), children's vocal ligaments are not fully functional until individuals are between 10 and 13 years of age. As Trollinger (2007) explains,

> Without a functioning vocal ligament, children produce most pitches for singing and speech by lengthening and thickening their vocal bands with their larynx in rest position. Since the bands are fairly short, they are limited in how much they can stretch, which results in a small pitch range for singing. (p. 20)

Many research studies have sought to define the pitches available to children in their comfortable singing ranges (Hedden, 2012). While no single range has been identified, there is agreement that this range has both a lower and an upper limit

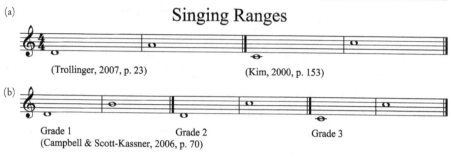

FIGURE 3.5

(Hedden, 2012). As well, the range appears to expand as children mature. As shown in Figure 3.5a, Trollinger (2007) identifies the vocal range for young children as from D above middle C to the A above, noting that this range corresponds with the pitches typically used by children when speaking. As well, this range fits well with the limited movements produced by the larynx of young children (Trollinger, 2007). Kim (2000) identifies the usual range for preschool children as the octave from middle C to C[1] (see Figure 3.5). Campbell and Scott-Kassner (2006) identify the typical vocal ranges for children in grades 1 to 3, noting how the range expands as the children's voices mature. In their opinion, the comfortable singing range for children in grade 1 is from D above middle C up to the B above. This expands to the seventh from D up to C for children in grade 2 and to the octave from middle C up to the C above for children in grade 3 (see Figure 3.5b). When modeling for young children, the pitches should be within this comfortable range. As well, young children should be monitored for signs of stress in singing (Trollinger, 2007) or sound production such as stretching their heads upwards to produce high tones and pointing their heads downwards when singing low tones. ⏵

Many children on the autism spectrum have limited verbal abilities. Early work in the classroom concentrates on helping these children explore their voices, keeping in mind that these children may be involved in group singing without the requirement to sing the words of songs with correct tones, rhythms, and expression. Many students are initially involved in singing activities through movement. As children gain more comfort with these experiences, they add vocalizations to these actions. This progression of interaction, from movement to vocalization added later is shown by the classroom vignette portrayed in text box 3.3. ⏵

Johnson (2002) proposes a hierarchy for vocal assessment in children with ASD. This hierarchy is presented with examples of how children on the autism spectrum may demonstrate the behaviors delineated in this hierarchy.

TEXT BOX 3.3
CLASSROOM VIGNETTE

Mrs. Greenspan observed that Phyllis enjoyed listening to her peers sing the song Engine, Engine, Number Nine (see Figure 3.6). Phyllis joined the class as they marched around the room in a train formation. After multiple experiences, Phyllis, who rarely vocalized, joined her peers by singing "choo choo" at the end of the chant to signify that the train had entered the station.

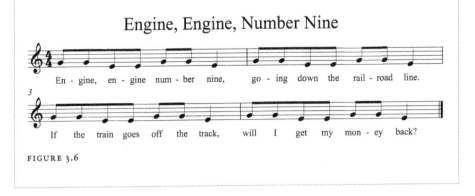

Engine, Engine, Number Nine

FIGURE 3.6

1. Students produce vocal sounds (by chance or on purpose)

Children may spontaneously produce vocal sounds during group singing experiences. Often these vocalizations are in the form of laughing or high pitched squeals that seem to reveal enjoyment of the singing experience. Other times squeals may become screams, indicating over stimulation. Teachers attend to such vocalizations, acknowledging enjoyment in some children and changing energy levels to help those who are overexcited.

2. Imitate vocal sounds (copy voice sounds or mouth sounds)

This second level, and those that follow, illustrate a child's conscious involvement in singing experiences. At this level children imitate vocal sounds. This could be sounds produced by the leader (e.g., the leader sings "hello" using a clear head voice, and the student responds). These responses could take many forms:

1. The student produces vocal sounds that are not recognized as words.
2. The student attempts to say "hello" with only part of the word distinguishable.
3. The student attempts to say "hello" but the word is only distinguishable by those familiar with his or her use of language.

4. The student sings "hello."

3. Sustain or repeat vocal sounds (play with the voice)

A student sings "hello" and everyone claps to acknowledge the student's success. The student smiles and repeats this word several times.

4. Imitate the musical contour of the sounds (copy the phrasing or melodic shape of sounds)

A student writes his or her name on the white board. The student uses a finger to trace the shape while using his or her voice to outline the contour of the letter.

5. Sing by imitating phrases (copy something sung by another person)

A student's favorite song is *Suogan* (see Figure 3.7). The teacher presents the song in four-beat phrases, providing time for the student to imitate each phrase before continuing the song. ▶

6. Sing to self (while working or playing)

A student loves the song *My favorite things* (Rodgers & Hammerstein, 2001). The student enjoys singing this song along with the music teacher. The student spontaneously sings his or her own version of this song outside of music class. While the melody and words do not exactly match the original, the song is unmistakable in the student's rendition.

7. Sing in presence of others (show independence, confidence)

A student enjoys clapping and swaying to the music as the leader and instructional assistants sing a repertoire of familiar songs in music class. The student has limited verbal abilities and chooses not to sing during class. The student's caregivers are

Suogan

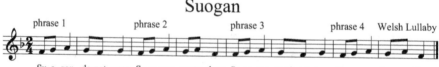

Su-o-gan, do not weep, Su-o-gan, go to sleep. Su-o-gan, moth-er's near, Su-o-gan, have no fear.

FIGURE 3.7

surprised when the student begins singing in school outside of music class. Through the school music experiences the student has acquired a repertoire of songs for which he or she knows the melody, rhythm, and all of the words.

8. Perform music [songs] in a classroom setting

A student has been in the same classroom setting since kindergarten. Now in grade 3, the student is able to sing songs with the rest of the class. Sometimes the student does not know all of the words so, for longer songs, the student claps the rhythm during the verses and sings the repeated choruses.

While these levels are described successively, they are not developmental in the sense that individuals graduate from one level to the next. Depending on the songs and the activities attached to these songs, children may be able to sing some songs with their peers (level 7) while, at the same time, acquire new repertoire by listening to what is sung by others and rehearse this material while involved in other activities at school or at home (level 6). As well, a child's responsiveness in music class depends on his or her disposition on a particular day. Educators are aware of how sensitive children with ASD are to changes in their regular routines, and allow them the space to respond in ways that best fit with what they are able to do. This is not an excuse for allowing children to display negative behaviors or to become a danger to themselves or to others. Rather, it is a reminder to respond to children with ASD as individuals, helping them to maximize their learning with and through music in ways that are appropriate at a particular time and in a particular space. This is illustrated in text box 3.4, through the story of Foster, a young boy whose willingness to participate in music class varies from day-to-day.

TEXT BOX 3.4
CLASSROOM VIGNETTE

Tuesday was a particularly good day for Foster. He interacted positively with caregivers and with his scheduled activities. He interacted positively with Mrs. Cooper in music class, responding to his name by singing an appropriate reply, and imitating phrases from known songs using the proper words, pitches, and rhythms. Wednesday was a difficult day for Foster. He struggled in all of his activities and did not want to attend music class. He did not respond to the teacher's greeting and did not participate in any of the singing activities. Sensing his frustration, Mrs. Cooper was happy to see Foster physically join the group by sitting in his assigned place and did not urge him to engage in the group's activities.

Echolalia

One of the primary determinants of ASD is an individual's difficulties in verbal communication. In general, children on the autism spectrum acquire speech by first repeating words in exact imitation of what they have heard in someone else's speech. Known as echolalia, this verbal strategy occurs in the speech of at least 85% of children with ASD who eventually gain the ability to speak (Rydell & Prizant, 1995). Some individuals with ASD acquire the ability to produce language independently by the time they are eight to ten years old. Other individuals rely on echolalic language into adolescence and adulthood (Prizant, 1987).

There are two types of echolalia, immediate and delayed. Immediate echolalia is evident when a child directly imitates what someone has said in the child's current surroundings. Delayed echolalia occurs when an individual repeats verbal sequences heard many hours, days, or weeks earlier (Prizant, 1983). In music classes, immediate echolalia often occurs when the teacher asks children to sing hello. For example, the teacher sings "hello Sarah" and the child returns the greeting by singing "hello Mrs. Morrison." This simple teaching strategy becomes complex when working with a child on the autism spectrum who, when given the greeting "hello Daniel," reverts to echolalic speech by singing "hello Daniel." Other times, children may find interest in a phrase sung or spoken by the leader. For example, the teacher introduces activities using a ball, by saying "the ball game." A child with echolalic speech may repeat the word *ball* every time he or she rolls the ball to a partner.

Teachers may observe delayed echolalia in music class when children spontaneously repeat phrases heard in prior situations. The content of delayed echolalia is often inappropriate in the current situation, for example, when a child suddenly recites dialogue from a movie that has seemingly no relationship to the present conversations or activities.

Research on echolalia reflects varying perspectives. Early research viewed echolalia as a "severe communication disorder" (Schreibman & Carr, 1978, p. 453) that hampered the development of functional speech. Given this view, caregivers were urged to discourage a child's propensity toward echolalic behaviors (Schreibman & Carr, 1978). Providing an alternate view, Prizant (1987) argues against echolalia as meaningless verbal repetition, maintaining, rather, that echolalia serves social functions, provides indications of comprehension, and supports the development of functional speech. From this perspective, by demonstrating echolalic behaviors a child may be "learning what can be accomplished through the production of speech, even though he may have limited linguistic knowledge to generate creative utterances" (Prizant, 1987, p. 82).

It is probable that teachers who work with children on the autism spectrum will observe echolalic behaviors in their students. Following Prizant (1987) these verbalizations should be encouraged as they may be a form of rehearsal for language that assists children in developing the ability to communicate with others through speech. Simiarly, song and singing can be used as a form of vocal rehearsal by providing students with opportunities to experiment with their voices by creating a variety of vocal sounds including sounds that are distinguishable as words. For example, students can use their voices to imitate contour, to practice creating words to accompany songs, and to imitate the words for songs as modeled by their teachers and other caregivers. A practical example of how a teacher may use music-based activities and songs to promote vocal behaviors is illustrated in text box 3.5.

To further understanding of echolalia in children with ASD, Prizant and Duchan (1981) examined how children with ASD use immediate echolalia when interacting with familiar adults. These researchers found that, in most instances, these verbalizations were accompanied by some level of comprehension and identified six interactive functions of echolalia: turn-taking, declarative, rehearsal, self-regulatory, yes-answer, and, request. I describe these functions for echolalic behaviors here, and add examples relevant to music education.

1. Turn-taking: During turn-taking activities the verbal echoes of children on the autism spectrum are used as "turn fillers in an alternating verbal exchange" (Prizant, 1983); the children's verbal responses may be accompanied by gazes towards a partner. For example, in music class, a child and partner play a drum. The child says the word *drum* when play transfers from one player to the other.

2. Declarative: During declarative interactions the child gestures toward a person or object while providing a verbal label through the use of echolalia. These verbalizations are directed toward the person or persons with whom the child is communicating. For example, the child points to a drum, while saying "drum" and gazing toward his or her partner in music class.

3. Rehearsal: These utterances, often whispered at low volume, are a form of echolalic thinking out loud that aids in the cognitive processing of these verbalizations. According to Prizant and Duchan (1981), "this strategy is analogous to what speakers do when attempting to learn a foreign language or when there is some distraction in the environment, that is, repeat the utterance to aid in comprehension" (p. 246). Rehearsal(s) of the word are followed by louder use of the word as a declarative interaction (see no. 2 above). For example, the child quietly rehearses the word *drum* before using the word to initiate interaction with a partner.

4. Self-regulatory: Similar to rehearsal, self-regulatory verbalizations appear to have a cognitive purpose. Unlike rehearsal, self-regulatory utterances do

TEXT BOX 3.5
CLASSROOM VIGNETTE

Mrs. Henderson uses a variety of activities to help grade 1 students experiment with their voices. She observes that these activities help children on the autism spectrum acquire vocal abilities and speech. As well, the activities help these children engage in activities with their peers. Marcel seems to enjoy the hot air balloon game in which the teacher moves some balloons and a basket across the classroom and the students use their voices to reflect the contour of the flight path. He experiments with his singing voice by improvising songs around his activities. For example, Mrs. Henderson heard him singing snippets of the song *Winter is Here* (Figure 3.8) while preparing to go home at the end of the school day. ▶

Echolalic rehearsal is seen in his initial attempts at singing. For example, Marcel repeats the word *farm* when singing the song *Old McDonald Had a Farm.* Mrs. Henderson does not interrupt these rehearsals, realizing that this process of rehearsal may help him to acquire speech.

Winter is Here

S. J. Scott

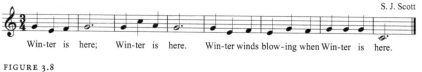

Win-ter is here; Win-ter is here. Win-ter winds blow-ing when Win-ter is here.

FIGURE 3.8

not lead to communicative interactions. Rather, self-regulatory verbalizations help a child direct his or her behaviors. These utterances are generally used in conjunction with motor activities. For example, a child is moving in circles while swinging a streamer. While engaged in this activity the child quietly repeats the word *round.*

5. Yes-answer: A yes answer denotes an echolalic (verbal) agreement to a prior utterance accompanied by a nonverbal indication of agreement. For example, the child says "drum." The teacher asks if the child wants the drum; the child's verbal response in the affirmative (yes) is accompanied by a gesture toward the drum.

6. Request: At this level the child indicates attention to people and/or objects in the surrounding environment. In educational settings, the child repeats some of the language used by the teacher (immediate echolalia) and adds

elements to indicate wants or needs. For example, the teacher asks: "What do you want"; the child responds: "What do you want drum."

These levels of echolalic behavior demonstrate that "modeling language in a context of active involvement and in synchrony with relevant action patterns is a powerful teaching strategy for autistic children" (Prizant, 1987, p. 85). Music based environments provide multiple opportunities for children on the autism spectrum to engage actively with others and, through these activities, to practice language through imitation. Engagement through music requires active involvement providing multiple opportunities to emphasize relationships between the child's use of imitative language and the immediate environment through demonstrative gestures (such as pointing) and actions with objects.

In general, music environments for early learners focus, in part, on the student's acquisition of in-tune singing. Many times song acquisition is taught through imitation as the children acquire a repertoire of known songs by imitating the teacher's vocal model. This is an ideal environment to promote echolalic speech, as all children, not just those on the autism spectrum, acquire skills through vocal (verbal) imitation. Providing appropriate vocal models and song literature are keys to providing an environment conducive to this learning.

Teachers' Vocal Models

Children imitate their teacher's actions. When singing, an educator provides a vocal model using a light head voice and pitches songs in a comfortable singing range in the hopes that children will imitate this model. In addition to performing songs with appropriate melodies and rhythms, the leader models the mood of the text using appropriate tempo and expression (such as dynamic levels). Enthusiasm is a key to motivating children's involvement in music. Teachers choose songs that they enjoy singing and express this enthusiasm through their facial expressions and body language. Their enthusiasm motivates students to take part in class activities by adding their own vocalizations to the teacher's or by moving in response to music. If a teacher feels unable to provide this model, he or she might consult instructional assistants as it is possible that one of these individuals may be able and willing to be the vocal leader during music class and at other times during the school day. Male teachers may prefer that female assistants lead the singing to provide a vocal model that reflects the children's singing range. Alternately, in inclusive settings, a student or a group of students who sing in tune may lead the singing.

While it is possible to replace live voices with recordings, recordings should be used sparingly. Recordings may add interesting accompaniments. However, many recordings (including those marketed specifically to children) are "over-orchestrated, with too many instruments, too many different kinds of instruments that force kids to overcompensate to be heard" (Trollinger, 2007, p. 24). In many contexts, a cappella singing or singing with an appropriate piano accompaniment provides the best opportunities for young children to develop their singing voices (Trollinger, 2007).

Choosing a Repertoire of Songs

Many general music programs for children are built around a repertoire of songs. In general, the same repertoire teachers use with typically developing students is suitable for use with individuals with ASD. This section provides a brief overview of criteria that teachers use when judging the usefulness and appropriateness of songs chosen to promote young children's vocal (and singing) development, from Kindergarten to approximately grade 3. Readers interested in more information about choosing song literature may wish to consult general music education textbooks such as Campbell and Scott-Kassner (2006) and Montgomery (2002).

MUSICAL CONSIDERATIONS

1. Range: The range of a song is the distance between the highest pitch and the lowest pitch. In order to promote the use of the child's head voice for singing, the range of songs should be within the range of the child's voice.
2. Scale: In music, the term *scale* is used to describe the organization of pitches, from lowest to highest, around a resting place (called a *tonal center*). The simplest songs may represent an incomplete scale by using only two notes. In general, the simplest complete scale used in children's songs is the 5-note pentatonic scale. This scale may center on the tonal center *do* (*do, re, mi, sol, la*) or the tonal center *la* (*la, do, re, mi, sol*). This scale is an ideal starting place for children's voices because it contains notes that step (e.g., *do* to *re*) or skip (e.g., *mi* to *sol*). More complicated songs use the major scale (*do, re, mi, fa, sol, la, ti, do*) or the natural minor scale (*la, ti, do, re, mi, fa, sol, la*).
3. Intervals: The term *interval* denotes the distance between two adjacent pitches. Simple children songs generally use pitches that repeat (the melody stays on the same line or space), move by step (the melody moves from a

line to the next space or from a space to the next line), or move by skip (the melody moves from a line to the next line or from a space to the next space). While melodies may move by leap (distances greater than a skip), these intervals are used sparingly as they are more difficult to sing in tune.

4. Rhythms: The terms *rhythms* or *rhythmic elements* denote the organization of sounds and silences over the basic pulse. Beginning song material generally employs the quarter note to represent the beat. The majority of rhythms represent the beat subdivided into two sounds of equal length (eighth notes) or the beat twice its usual length (half note). More complicated rhythms are added as students gain facility with these.

5. Meter: The term *meter* denotes the organization of the beat around regular groupings of accented and unaccented beats. The songs referenced in this publication are generally organized around the quarter note in groups of 2 (2/4 meter), 3 (3/4 meter) and 4 (4/4 meter). Each grouping is called a *measure*.

6. Length: A song's *length* is generally described as the number of *measures*. The first songs that children learn generally range from 8 to 16 measures in length. Longer songs are added as the students' attention spans lengthen. Older children especially enjoy songs that contain several verses with repeated choruses.

These guidelines directed the selection of songs referred to in this publication. These songs are easily accessible to young children and are therefore appropriate for those working with children in a variety of educational environments, including inclusive classrooms and groupings of children with special needs, such as those with ASD. These songs, as well as others that adhere to these principles, provide a basis for helping children to acquire singing ability. As well, these songs provide multiple avenues for interaction through music.

TEXTS

In choosing song literature, educators assess the text. Several questions guide this assessment:

1. Is the text developmentally appropriate?

Texts must be developmentally appropriate for the students. Young children tend to enjoy songs that suggest accompanying movements (e.g., *Engine Engine Number Nine*). They also appreciate songs about personal experiences (e.g., *Rain, Rain, Go*

Away). Older children like songs about nature. In general, children of all ages enjoy songs that mark the changes of the seasons and that celebrate holidays.

Choosing developmentally appropriate resources is especially important when working with children on the autism spectrum. Teachers might be tempted to choose songs more appropriate for younger children in an attempt to help those who struggle with language. It is more desirable to choose songs that are age-appropriate so that students are motivated to be engaged in the songs and the activities that accompany the songs. This guideline should be applied with discretion. While it might not be feasible to construct an entire music program for ten-year-old children around songs for younger individuals, it does no harm to maintain a few of the children's favorite songs from earlier years in their current repertoire.

2. Does the song lend itself to visual imagery and/or drama?

Given the penchant of children on the autism spectrum for visual understanding, it is advantageous to choose songs that lend themselves to visual imagery and/or drama. Songs about animals may be accompanied with pictures or objects that represent the animals in question (e.g., *The cat came back* [Slavin, 1992] is accompanied by a toy cat); songs that tell a story may be acted out by children who take on the roles of the characters (e.g., the song *The Farmer in the Dell* [Figure 3.9]). This story is illustrated in the picture book by the same name (O'Brien, 2000). ⊙

The Farmer in the Dell

Traditional Game Song

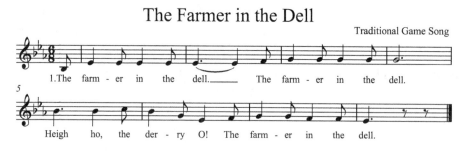

1. The farm-er in the dell.___ The farm-er in the dell.
Heigh ho, the der-ry O! The farm-er in the dell.

2. The farmer takes a wife.
3. The wife takes a child.
4. The child takes a nurse.
5. The nurse takes a cow.
6. The cow takes a dog.
7. The dog takes a cat.
8. The cat takes a rat.
9. The rat takes the cheese.
10. The cheese stands alone.

FIGURE 3.9

3. Do the words of the text fit with the melody and rhythm?

This may not be a concern when working with folk songs such as those included in this book. These songs have been sung for generations and, through oral transmission, lyrics have been established to fit with the structure of the music. This generalization only holds when songs are sung in their original language. Translated materials should be reviewed to see that the syllables of the translations work with the melody and rhythm of the song.

4. Does the song contain repetition in words and music?

Many children's songs display repetition in the musical structure and/or the words. This helps students to be able to sing the song in tune and to acquire the ability to reproduce the words.

LEADING SONGS

Teachers may wish to think about the following considerations when preparing to lead songs.

1. Beginning Pitch

Many teachers are able to establish a beginning pitch through a mental rehearsal of the piece (that is, performing the song in their head without singing it aloud). This skill develops with practice over time. Teachers unable to choose a beginning pitch in this manner often use a musical instrument such as a keyboard, a recorder, or a xylophone, to provide the first pitch of the song.

2. Tonality

To lead group singing, the teacher needs to have a sense of the tonality of a piece. Is it a major tonality with a resting place at *do* or is it a minor tonality with a resting place at *la*? The teacher may establish the tonality by singing a foundational chord (often *do, mi, sol* in a major key or *la, do, mi* in a minor key). Teachers who are unable to perform this task through a silent rehearsal of the piece often use a musical instrument such as keyboard, recorder, or xylophone to provide this aural information.

3. Meter

Meter guides the rendition of accented and unaccented beats in performance. In folk material, these patterns of accented and unaccented beats fit with the words of the piece and portray its character accurately. Teachers should perform songs in a meter that portrays the natural accents of the words. For example, sing a song such as *Star Light, Star Bright* in both 2/4 and 4/4 meter with an emphasis on the first beat of each measure (see Figure 3.10). ▶

When doing so, take note of how the accents at the beginning of each measure in 2/4 meter provide a more natural emphasis for the text than 4/4 meter. For example, the text has a better flow with a metric accent each time the word *star* is sung (2/4) than with an accent only on the first *star* in 4/4 meter. The same is true for *wish I may, wish I might*. *Wish* is accented each time it is sung in 2/4 meter; in 4/4 meter this word is given a metric accent only once.

4. Style (tempo/dynamics)

When leading group singing, teachers establish an appropriate tempo for the piece before beginning to sing. The chosen tempo portrays the style of the song: for example, a lullaby such as *All Through the Night* (Figure 3.11) is sung at a slower tempo than an active song such as *This Old Man* (Figure 3.12). Similarly, the dynamics suit the style of the piece. So, *All Through the Night* would be sung more quietly than *This Old Man*. When singing loudly, children generally need reminders not to sing (or shout) as loudly as possible but to use their proper singing voices. ▶ ▶

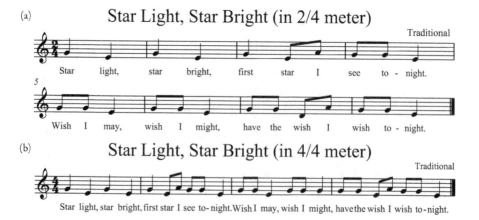

FIGURE 3.10

All Through the Night

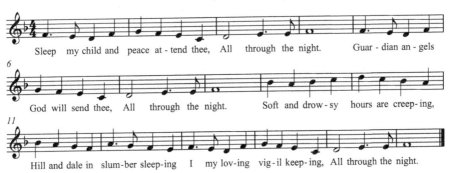

Sleep my child and peace at-tend thee, All through the night. Guar-dian an-gels God will send thee, All through the night. Soft and drow-sy hours are creep-ing, Hill and dale in slum-ber sleep-ing I my lov-ing vig-il keep-ing, All through the night.

FIGURE 3.11

This Old Man

Traditional

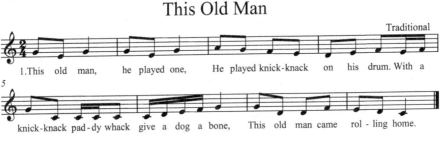

1.This old man, he played one, He played knick-knack on his drum. With a knick-knack pad-dy whack give a dog a bone, This old man came rol-ling home.

2. shoe; 3. knee; 4. door; 5. hive; 6. sticks; 7. up in heaven; 8. gate; 9. all the time

FIGURE 3.12

TEACHING SONGS BY ROTE

Songs are generally taught to young children by rote. The following describes this approach:

1. Teacher sings the song.
2. Teacher leads students in a discussion about the song using visuals such as stuffed toys or other props to add visual information to the discussion. These visuals help students to understand the song and adds motivation and excitement to the process of song (and singing) acquisition.
3. Teacher sings the first phrase of the song.
4. Students imitate teacher by repeating the first phrase.
5. If students sing this phrase correctly, teacher sings the next phrase and students repeat. If students do not sing the first phrase correctly, teacher may sing that phrase again and ask students to repeat it. Teacher may use a hand to show the contour of the phrase and the length of the rhythms as this will assist students in manipulating their voices.

6. Teacher continues by teaching each phrase in this manner.

7. Once students have learned the whole song phrase by phrase, teacher goes to the beginning of the song and asks students to imitate larger sections, perhaps by grouping phrases into pairs. Teacher asks students to repeat small segments to correct any mistakes immediately.

8. This process is repeated with large segments of the song until students are able to sing the whole piece.

WHOLE SONG APPROACH

I had been a music teacher for several years before I began teaching children on the autism spectrum. I was accustomed to teaching songs by rote using the process described above. The first time I taught a group of children with special educational needs, I began by singing a song and sharing some background information about the song. It became evident very quickly that teaching songs phrase-by-phrase was not an effective way to introduce songs to children who did not speak. In this context, I found the whole song approach more effective.

Using the whole song approach, the teacher chooses a group of songs with which he or she would like the students to become familiar. During music time the teacher plans a singing segment in which he or she sings selections from this group of songs. Students are involved in the singing activities through movements. They are encouraged to hum or vocalize along with the singer, even if they are unable to sing the correct pitches or words. Once children are familiar with the names and topics of the songs, the teacher shows them visuals representing these songs. This increases their involvement in music class as they are asked to choose the songs they sing. Through repeated involvement with the whole song, students gain familiarity with its musical structure and the text. Over time students begin to sing words or whole phrases of these songs. Sometimes the words represent the use of echolalia when, for example, a student repeats the word *springtime* while the teacher sings *The twelve days of springtime* (Rose & Armstrong-Ellis, 2009). Eventually some students are able to sing a whole song or group of songs, acquiring this repertoire through the whole song approach. This process is illustrated in text box 3.6.

Vocal Experiences for Children on the Autism Spectrum

Teachers try to create educational environments that support children on the autism spectrum as those children build on their natural tendencies toward music, learning to interact with music experiences in ways that are appropriate for their levels

TEXT BOX 3.6
CLASSROOM VIGNETTE

William is interested in sounds. He looks toward the window when he hears birds chirping, he looks toward the door when he hears teachers talking in the hallway, and he bends his head toward the computer speakers, amazed by the music that emits from them. He listens to the recording that accompanies the book *We all go traveling by* (Roberts & Bell, 2003) every day. When the class sings the song, Mrs. Choo models the same pitches as sung on the recording because she knows these are the pitches that William uses and does not want to confuse him by using different pitches. Words from the song (e.g., *school bus, truck, train, bike, boat, plane, car*) become vocabulary key words, helping William to make the link between singing these words in the song and using these words in speech.

of engagement. In the following section ways in which to involve students in music experiences through songs and singing are examined. Additional strategies for helping children to sing in tune are found in textbooks for teaching elementary classroom music such as Boyer and Rozmajzl (2012) and Herrold (2001).

MOTIVATION

Children with ASD are motivated by music. Teachers of music may build on this propensity by personalizing music experiences. Three strategies are described:

A. Personalizing a greeting
B. Personalizing songs
C. Language as song (sung speech)

Personalizing a greeting

In general, individuals with ASD thrive on routine. Establishing a routine in music class helps these students feel safe within their school environments. One way to establish routine is to begin each class session with the same song. Students in the class might be motivated by a song tailored toward their educational context. This is demonstrated with the *Music Class Cheer Song* illustrated in Figure 3.13. ▶

This song may be adapted for many classrooms by exchanging the words "grade 2" with a word or words appropriate to a particular group of students, such as "play school community." As well, the place name may be substituted with words suited

Music Class Cheer Song

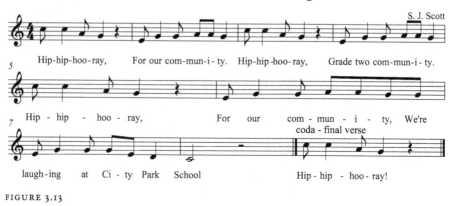

Hip-hip-hoo-ray, For our com-mun-i-ty. Hip-hip-hoo-ray, Grade two com-mun-i-ty.

Hip - hip - hoo - ray, For our com - mun - i - ty, We're

laugh-ing at Ci - ty Park School Hip-hip - hoo-ray!

FIGURE 3.13

to particular contexts. Children show enjoyment and appreciation for this song by clapping and moving as it is sung.

Personalizing songs

Personalizing songs motivates students. Names and descriptors may be included in songs and photographs may be added to illustrate the activities the lyrics describe. For example, in the song *Fall is on its Way* (Figure 3.14), a second verse, *Little boys go out to play*, corresponds to the picture.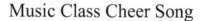

Subsequent verses are composed about particular students and the activities in which they like to engage, with photographs used to personalize the songs further. It is important to adhere to school procedures and policies when taking photographs of children. In some schools taking photographs of children and showing these in music class may not be allowed; in other cases the teacher may need signed consent. In many cases, photographs taken for class activities may not be shown outside of the class.

Language as song (sung speech)

Some students with ASD respond more readily to language presented as song than to spoken language. This observation was explored by Kern, Wolery, and Aldridge (2007) who examined the effects of songs on the behaviors of two children with autism by using a composed song to outline the classroom's morning routine. These researchers found that "the songs . . . assisted the children in entering the classroom, greeting the teacher and/or peers and engaging in play" (Kern et al., p. 1264). This phenomenon is illustrated in text box 3.7.

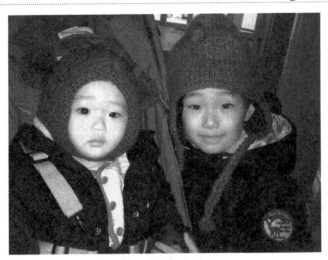

Fall is on its Way

S. J. Scott

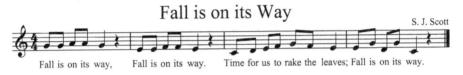

Fall is on its way,   Fall is on its way.   Time for us to rake the leaves; Fall is on its way.

FIGURE 3.14

Teachers may apply this research finding in their classrooms by replacing spoken language with song fragments (either pre-composed or improvised). The use of these song fragments mirrors that of verbal interactions:

1. To gain a student's attention (Figure 3.15)
2. To inform students of expectations (Figure 3.16)
3. To reward successes (Figure 3.17) ▶ ▶ ▶

Teachers who work with children on the autism spectrum may choose to experiment with song fragments to replace speech and observe how their students respond to this technique. They may find that the use of sung speech is an effective way to gain a student's attention and engagement for class activities.

PITCH DISCRIMINATION

The ability to discriminate and remember melodic sequences (the contour of successive pitches) is a precursor to accurate pitch production. The following activities provide students opportunities to demonstrate their understanding of pitches and pitch contour without relying on speech.

Sung Speech

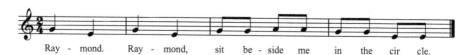

FIGURE 3.15 Sung Speech for Gaining a Student's Attention

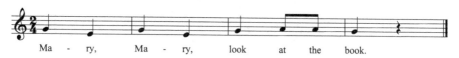

FIGURE 3.16 Sung Speech for Informing Expectations

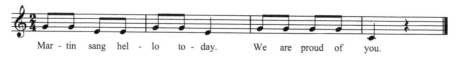

FIGURE 3.17 Sung Speech for Rewarding Success

Kazoo

The teacher produces sounds with a kazoo and asks the children to use movements
to illustrate the contours of the sounds

Voice

Using the voice is an effective way for teachers to interact with individual students.
For example, a teacher may stand in front of a particular student and use his or her
voice to reflect this student's actions. This becomes a game as the student takes the

lead by creating high and low movements which the teacher mirrors with his or her voice. While the kazoo may also be used in this way, vocal sounds alone may be more effective with this variation of the activity because there is no instrument between the teacher and the students.

PITCH PRODUCTION

Auditory awareness and discrimination provides a foundation for language development. This begins with experimentation, such as the production of vocal sounds, and may progress to the spontaneous use of particular words or phrases to accompany familiar songs. Five strategies for encouraging vocal production are outlined below: call and response, outlining contour, playing kazoo, songs without words, and songs and language development.

Call and response

Many teachers begin music sessions with call and response activities in which the leader sings "hello" and the students provide their own "hello" in response. Props such as toy microphones or puppets can be used to motivate the students to respond. A typical interaction is illustrated in Figure 3.18. ▶

The following descriptions portray the behaviors demonstrated by children on the autism spectrum when attempts are made to engage them in this activity:

1. Student looks away and does not acknowledge the leader.
2. Student looks in the direction of the leader but does not seem to acknowledge that person.
3. Student does not look at the leader's face but there does seem to be recognition for the adult; child may reach for the microphone.
4. Student may reach for microphone and produce vocal sounds that match the leader's pitch.
5. Student may reach for microphone and attempt to speak words in response.
6. Student sings "hello" into the microphone.

Typical Greeting

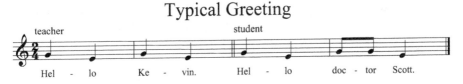

FIGURE 3.18

Possible Greeting for Student with Echolalia

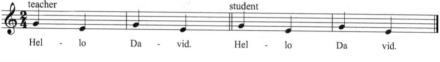

FIGURE 3.19

This strategy may reveal challenges when used with students with immediate echo-lalia. In this case, the child might not change the greeting to reflect his or her point of view. This sort of exchange is illustrated in Figure 3.19. ▶

This interchange reveals the difficulties that children with ASD have in perceiving themselves in relation to others (Hobson & Lee, 1999; Williams, Whiten, & Singh, 2004). To assist with this understanding, the following exchange among the music teacher (Dr. Scott), an instructional assistant (IA; Mrs. Penner), and the student (David) may be helpful:[1]

1. Teacher points to self and sings: "Dr. Scott"
2. Teacher points at IA and sings: "Mrs. Penner"
3. Teacher points at child and sings: "David"
4. Teacher points to IA and sings: "Hello Mrs. Penner"
5. IA points to teacher and sings: "Hello Dr. Scott"
6. Teacher points to David and sings: "Hello David"
7. Teacher points to self while prompting David to sing: "Hello Dr. Scott"

A child may need time and space to provide a response and to practice this task. The teacher is sensitive to the child's needs and observes the child's behaviors while using this strategy. If the child becomes agitated or disengages he or she is letting the teacher know that it is time to move to the next activity.

Vocalizing contour

Vocalizing contours is a motivating way for students to practice tone production. As well, this activity provides avenues for students who have difficulties forming words to demonstrate their ability to perceive and produce pitch. This activity also provides students with opportunities to follow directions and to show understand-ing of some of the terms applied to contour such as high, low, getting higher, and getting lower. Two ways to approach vocalizing contours are described: "alphabet" and "the fish in the sea."

Alphabet

Students vocalize the shapes of letters of the alphabet. A suggested procedure follows:

1. A student approaches the white board.
2. The student draws the letter at the beginning of his or her name (e.g., G for George).
3. The teacher or student traces the outline of this letter and the student vocalizes the contour. For example, a student named Michael prints a capital M on the board. The teacher begins to trace this letter beginning at the lower left corner. As the teacher traces a part of the letter that ascends, Michael produces ascending vocal sounds; as the teacher traces a part of the letter that descends, Michael produces descending vocal sounds. Another student, Joyce, prints a capital J. The teacher begins to trace this letter at the top. As the teacher traces the letter downward, Joyce produces decendng vocal sounds; as the curve of the J ascends, Joyce produces ascending vocal sounds.
4. The teacher or student traces the outline of this letter and all members of the class vocalize the shape of this outline.

Fish in the sea

The teacher shows a simple drawing of the sea on a whiteboard with a wavy line toward the top to show the waves and some rocks, plants, and sea creatures at the bottom of the picture. The teacher produces a cardboard drawing of a fish. A fish puppet is also an effective prop for this activity. The teacher manipulates the fish so it swims in the sea. The children's vocalizations imitate the contour in the movements of the fish.[2]

Kazoo

Kazoos are an inexpensive way to provide children on the autism spectrum with a melodic instrument. If possible, each child and instructional assistant are assigned an instrument. Labels with the player's name may be attached to the bottom of the instruments so that individuals can be given the same instrument each time the class meets. Each instrument is placed inside its own plastic bag for easy distribution prior to class and collection at the end of class. This helps address issues around the sanitary use of instruments that children place in their mouths and also gives the students a sense of ownership as a particular kazoo becomes their instrument.

Playing the kazoo

It takes time, patience, and modeling to teach children how to create vocal sounds using kazoos but the enjoyment they gain once they master the process is well worth the effort involved. Suggested strategies for teaching the kazoo include:

1. Provide the child with an instrument. The teacher faces the child and vocalizes with the instrument. The teacher then asks the child to play his or her instrument. If the child is disengaged or does not understand, step 1 is repeated in future sessions. If the child attempts to make a sound but is unable to vocalize in a way appropriate to the instrument, move to step 2. If the child vocalizes an appropriate sound on the kazoo, move to the next heading, experimentation.
2. The teacher hums without the instrument and asks the child to hum. The teacher then plays the instrument again and asks the child to hum into the instrument.

My first attempt at teaching kazoo was not successful. The students looked at me with puzzled faces and did not understand what they were being asked to do. I put the kazoos aside until the next year. When the kazoos were reintroduced, one of the students was immediately able to play and another student was able to vocalize with the instrument by the following week. This emphasizes how the readiness of children to participate in music is an important guide in planning music-based activities.

When working in inclusive environments, the teacher might start by providing kazoos to small groups of children and, over time, work with all individuals in small groups so that eventually everyone forms a kazoo choir.

EXPERIMENTATION. Once students are able to produce appropriate sounds using the kazoo, they need time to experiment with the instrument by producing different types of sounds:

- High sounds
- Low sounds
- Fast Sounds
- Slow Sounds
- Contoured Sounds (variations of high and low)

This is an important step in creating music as children have opportunities to see first-hand what they can do with this instrument. As well, provided that students play the instrument in an appropriate manner, whatever tones they produce are correct. This creates a positive avenue for celebrating individual students' successes.

IMITATIVE IMPROVISATIONS. Spaces for children to experiment with kazoos are coupled with interactions between teacher and student using imitative improvisations. In this activity, the teacher produces a four-beat motive on the kazoo and pauses for the student to reply. Responses take many forms:

- Student disengages, does not look at the teacher and does not provide a reply on the kazoo.
- Student may or may not look at the teacher; student produces a reply that is either shorter or longer than that of the teacher.
- Student may look at the teacher; student produces a reply the same length as that of the teacher.
- Student may look at the teacher; student's reply imitates some of the teacher's pitches and rhythms.
- Student may look at the teacher; student's reply imitates the teacher's pitches and rhythms.

This is not necessarily a hierarchy with a child graduating from one level of behavior to the next. The child's ability to perform at one level or another is dependent, in part, on that child's behaviors on particular days.

Choksy (1999) suggests that in question and answer activities the teacher's motives are derived from the patterns in the child's known song material. This ensures that the resulting musical conversations fit within the context of the student's prior musical experiences.

Songs and kazoos
ECHO SONGS. As the name suggests, echo songs are structured in two parts with a leader and a follower or followers. The leader sings a phrase and the followers repeat what has been sung. Using echo songs to involve children on the autism spectrum in music class by vocalizing with kazoos is profiled through the song *Down by the Bay* (Figure 3.20).

Down by the Bay is often performed as an echo song with the leader singing a phrase and the followers producing the echo. This is shown in the notation presented in Figure 3.20 with the leader singing the notation on the top staff and the

Down by the Bay

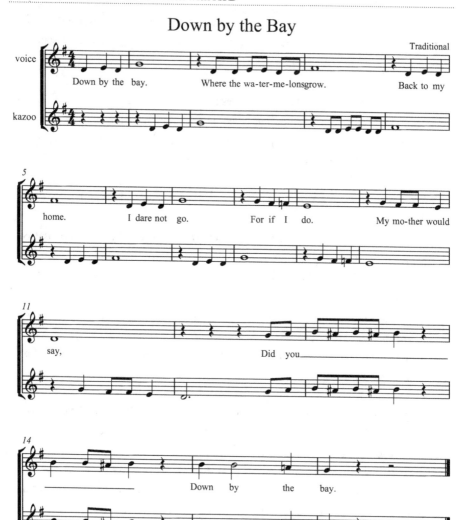

FIGURE 3.20

echo notated on the bottom staff. Where straight lines are shown in place of lyrics the group inserts a phrase. These are often nonsense words describing animals, such as:

Have you ever seen a bear, combing his hair.
Have you ever seen a llama, eating a banana.

The leader may also insert phrases that incorporate the children's names, such as:

Have you ever seen a Jen, writing with a pen.
Have you ever seen a Mike, riding his bike.

Changes in the words often require slight adaptations in the melody and rhythm so that the lyrics fit with the song.

A teacher may wish to involve students with this song using the following process:

1. The teacher sings the parts of the song designated for a leader and plays the echoes on a kazoo.
2. After the students are familiar with the song, they are guided to vocalize the echoes on kazoos.

Achieving the second step in this procedure may require practice. Some students may immediately understand when they are to play the kazoo, while others need varying degrees of assistance. For example, the teacher might use body language to indicate when the children are to play and when they should listen. Alternately, students with verbal ability could sing the song and those who are unable to speak could add the echoed phrases on kazoos.

SONGS WITH SIMPLE REPEATED SYLLABLES

It is important for teachers to support individual students' efforts to verbalize during singing experiences. A range of verbal behavior is possible:

- Laughing
- Non-speaking sounds that often reflect the teacher's pitches
- Sounds that resemble words but that cannot be identified by others
- Words in the child's vocabulary
- Words of the song

While children are able to vocalize with any song, songs containing simple, repeated syllables are particularly useful for encouraging students with ASD to sing along with their peers. Individuals with ASD may vocalize during portions of these songs using the expected syllables or inventing their own words. Through

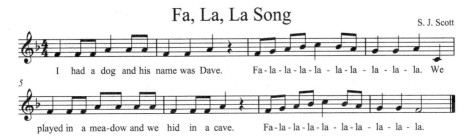

FIGURE 3.21

continued experience, some students improve the clarity with which they reproduce the repeated syllables and/or the words in the songs. They may also increase the number of phrases they vocalize, singing not only the repeated syllables but other words or phrases in a particular song. I illustrate this with a *Fa, La, La* song composed to encourage vocal participation from students with ASD (see Figure 3.21). This is a simple four-phrase song, with phrases 1 and 3 providing a narrative and phrases 2 and 4 providing a simple refrain on the syllables fa, la, la. Given the simplicity of the lyrics, students with ASD may be motivated to participate vocally by joining peers on phrases 2 and 4 by replicating the fa, la, la syllables or by creating their own syllables for the duration of these phrases. Over time, some students are better-able to produce the fa-la-la syllables accurately; others may begin to replicate the words in phrases 1 and 3. Teachers and/or students may create their own verses to extend this song. In a similar vein, children enjoy singing the *la* sections of the song portrayed in the book *Sing* (Raposo & Lichtenheld, 2013). Students may also be motivated to join their peers in singing the repeated E-I-E-I-O pattern in the song Old MacDonald had a Farm (see Figure 3.22). ▶ ▶

SONGS AND LANGUAGE DEVELOPMENT

Lim (2012) describes using songs and singing to promote interverbal communication in children on the autism spectrum. According to Lim, interverbal communication is "a type of expressive language in which a word or phrase evokes another word or phrase by cueing or prompting, but the cue is not identical to the response (target word/phrase)" (Lim, 2012, p. 126). In music class, teachers may promote interverbal communications using songs that are illustrated as books. To implement this technique, the teacher chooses a singing book with which a child has gained familiarity through repeated listening. The teacher highlights words at the ends of phrases by

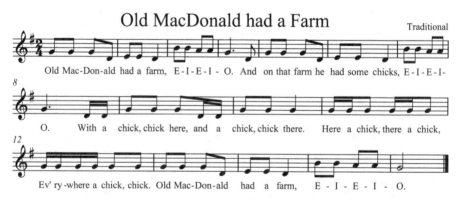

FIGURE 3.22

singing the phrases and pausing before the last word and waiting for the child to complete the sentence.

Using the book *Sleep, baby, sleep* (Weidner, 2009), the teacher sings:

Sleep, baby, _____. (missing word: *sleep*)

If the child completes the phrase by singing or speaking the missing word, in this case *sleep*, the teacher proceeds to the next phrase:

Your father tends the _____. (missing word: *sheep)*

This interaction may continue throughout the book. If the child does not sing or speak the missing word, the teacher sings this word to complete the phrase and continues with the next phrase. After the child is able to sing the book in this manner, the teacher may extend the child's language use by asking him or her to replace the final two words of the phrase:

Sleep, _____. (missing words: *baby, sleep*)

Eventually, using this chaining technique, the child may sing the entire song. With time and practice the interverbal skills acquired and practiced through music may transfer to verbal skills in other contexts (Lim, 2012).

This is a difficult task. Not only must the child attend to the presentation of the book, he or she must generate target words or phrases and time these verbalizations to fit with the beat and rhythm of the song (Lim, 2012). Lim (2012) uses this technique in her work as a music therapist. This procedure may also be used by music teachers, in collaboration with a child's education team. The procedure may also be used by members of the child's education team who teach through music. This approach may seem well suited only to one-on-one interactions. However, it may be adapted to whole class settings with all students, or small groups of students, adding the missing word or words at the end of the phrases. The introduction of this technique could take place in the whole class [inclusion] setting and then be followed up with one-on-one interventions. Alternately, the one-on-one work could precede the use of this strategy in a whole class situation, thereby providing a child on the autism spectrum with the background and practice needed to complete this task along with his peers in inclusive educational settings.

PICTURE BOOKS BASED ON SONGS

A picture book can take many forms. It can be a wordless book, which tells a story solely through illustrations. It can be an illustrated book, in which the words carry most of the message, but illustrations either depict what is stated in the text or decorate the page. It can be a picture storybook, in which a tale is told through a combination of illustrations and text, each amplifying the other to create a unified whole. (Temple, Martinez, Yokota, & Naylor, 2002, p. 177)

As Temple et al. note, there are many ways to define the term *picture book*. In this section, discussion is limited to picture books in which the text and illustrations represent songs. These are denoted here as *singing books*.

Many children on the autistic spectrum are visual learners (American Psychiatric Association [APA], 2013). They have difficulty interpreting the meaning of words. In some instances responses to requests seem delayed because it takes children on the autism spectrum longer to interpret verbal instructions than their typically developing peers. By using singing books, teachers provide these students with an additional medium from which to understand the meaning of the songs presented in music class.

Traditional English language children's songs such as *Over in the meadow* (Wadsworth & Vojtech, 2002) have found new audiences when portrayed as singing books. Modern interpretations of traditional English language songs, such as *Pete the cat: The wheels on the bus* (Dean, 2013), motivate students by linking content from literature (the *Pete the Cat* book series) to the music classroom. Songs such as *The animal boogie* (Harter, 2000) and *Up, up, up* (Reed & Oldfield, 2010) are newly-composed songs released in tandem with picture books that provide a visual landscape for the song. Finally, songs from popular culture have been released as picture books. Examples of this are Starr and Cort's (2014) *Octopus's garden*, Yarrow and Lipton's (2007) *Puff, the magic dragon*, and Yarrow and Sweet's (2009) *Day is done*. An annotated bibliography of singing books, including a description of the content and structure of each book and an explanation of how teachers might use these resources is posted on the companion website. ▶

Choosing singing books

Factors to consider when choosing singing books are described below.

1. Is the subject matter concrete?

Concrete subject matter makes the topic more tangible for the students. For example, the book *Ten in the bed* (Stott, 2010) may involve the presentation of ten toy creatures (e.g., birds, animals) with one character taken away at the end of each verse to represent the story of the song.

2. Can the book clarify and expand students' understanding of their and other's experiences?

Picture books can help students to make sense of the day-to-day activities in their lives. For example, in *Here we go round the mulberry bush* (Fatus & Penner, 2007), the verses take the children through the activities they undertake as they prepare to go to school (e.g., brush teeth, comb hair). In Barnwell's *No Windows in My Nana's House* (1998), the experiences of a young girl may reflect the experience of the students or may provide an avenue to explore understanding of others.

3. Is the text portrayed as complete sentences, or, in music, as complete phrases?

A sentence-by-sentence or phrase-by-phrase format helps teachers to coordinate the turning of the pages with the performance of the song. As well, the students are better able to maintain their focus on the book and the song if the pages are turned at regular intervals in keeping with the phrases of the song.

4. Length

The length of the story should hold the students' interest. Pay attention to repetition as children are able to attend to longer books if the story has a predictable, repetitive structure. For example, *Old MacDonald had a farm* (no author, 2008) is created around a series of verses which feature numerous animals. The verse ends with a listing of all previous animals mentioned to that point in the book. Similarly, in *The farmer in the dell* (O'Brien, 2000) all words are the same except for the particular character featured in each stanza.

Some books are structured so that one or two pages portray a complete stanza, To illustrate, the book *Out on the prairie* (Taylor & Stephens, 2002) is a counting song in which each stanza portrays a particular mother animal with her baby or babies, such as antelope, badgers, and hawks. When using a book such as this, teachers may choose to present only a portion of the story in a particular class session, observing the students' body language to determine when the students are losing focus or interest.

5. Sequencing

The story portrayed in a singing book should unfold in a logical sequence of events. For example, in Vetter's (2009) depiction of *Down by the station*, the story begins at the station in the morning and ends back at the station at the end of the day.

6. Illustrations

Illustrations must clearly portray the story. The illustrations should enhance the words of the text and not detract from or obscure their meaning. There needs to be clear agreement between the text on the page and the illustrations.

7. Variety

When taken as a whole, the singing books used in a particular classroom can reflect a variety of songs including visual portrayals of traditional songs (*The wheels on the bus*, Kovalski, 1987), modern remakes of traditional songs (*Knick knack paddy whack* [also known as *This Old Man*], Engel & Songs, 2008), newly composed songs released in tandem with a book (*We all go traveling by*, Roberts & Bell, 2003) and; songs from popular culture (*Blowin' in the wind*, Dylan & Muth, 2011).

8. Diversity

It is important to use resources that depict children of multiple ethnicities. This is highlighted in many resources published by Barefoot books including *Here we go round the mulberry bush* (Fatus & Penner, 2007) with pictures that show how children in Europe, Mali, India, and China prepare for their day and the book *If you're happy and you know it* (McQuinn & Fatus, 2009) with illustrations of children from around the world in traditional dress. Many children's books, such as *The animal boogie* (Harter, 2000) and *Octopus's garden* (Starr & Cort, 2014) depict children with physical challenges.

Using singing books
Preparation
Before introducing a singing book to students, the teacher performs the book aloud to an imaginary audience and decides how to portray the song with appropriate tempo and dynamics. The teacher also learns how the text corresponds to the beat, rhythm, meter, and melody of the song, making note of how the accents of the words flow with the accented and unaccented beats of the song. The teacher also learns how the syllables of the words correspond with the rhythm of the song. Finally, the teacher practices turning the pages while singing the song to ensure that handling the book does not hinder performance of the song.

If presenting a modern adaptation of a traditional English language song, look for any changes in the text or music that affect the performance of the song. Similarly,

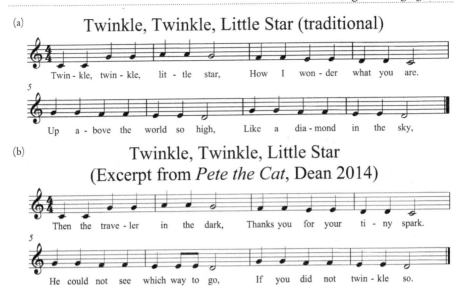

FIGURE 3.23

newly composed songs released as picture books should be assessed to ascertain the relation of the text with the music. For example, the first phrase of the song *Twinkle, Twinkle, Little Star* employs simple quarter note and half note patterns. Newly-composed verses in the book *Pete the cat: Twinkle, twinkle, little star* (Dean 2014) require adjustments to the traditional rhythm (see Figure 3.23). While not difficult to incorporate into performance, such changes should be practiced before the piece is presented to the students. ▶

Many publishers include compact discs with recordings of the songs. As well, recorded versions of many of the songs portrayed in picture books may be accessed from electronic sources. Teachers may use the recorded sources to help them to learn to perform the songs. These resources may also be used in the class as the instrumental accompaniments add another dimension to the music experience. I sometimes find that the tempi of recorded versions are too fast for my students, especially if they are just becoming familiar with the songs and the accompanying books. I tend to sing the songs and present the books using tempi that do not overwhelm the students, and introduce a recording after students are familiar with a particular singing book.

Performance

The teacher might introduce a book to students by showing them the cover illustration and leading a short discussion about what the book is about. I introduce a new singing book to the students by singing the song while showing the illustrations.

After children gain familiarity with the singing book, I invite students to become engaged in this musical experience through multiple avenues such as singing, moving, and playing instruments.

SINGING. Songs with repetitive structures promote students' involvement as vocalizers and/or singers. For example, in *Old MacDonald had a farm* (no author, 2008), children may add sounds to represent the animals; in *The cat came back* (Slavin, 1992) students often join in the repeated chorus, sometimes with their own vocalizations and other times adding words or portions of words.

MOVING. Movement is a natural outlet for involvement through music. For example, lullabies, such as *Hush little baby* (Frazee, 1999), provide a natural stimulus for rocking motions; lively songs, such as *The animal boogie* (Harter, 2000), provide an avenue for full body movements that imitate the animals portrayed.

PLAYING INSTRUMENTS. Students with limited verbal abilities gain involvement in singing through playing instruments. Rhythm sticks and drums create avenues for playing the beat to accompany songs such as *Knick knack paddy whack* (Engel & Songs, 2008) and *The seals on the bus* (Hort, 2000). Books such as *Old MacDonald had a workshop* (Shulman, 2002), provide an opportunity for instrument playing as leader, students, or leader and students in collaboration choose instruments to portray the tools used in the story (e.g., saw, drill, hammer)

Summary

Singing books are ideal resources for merging aural (singing) and visual (illustrations) information into integrated wholes. These resources are well suited for students with ASD, as these learners often rely on visual information when seeking to understand their environment. Singing books help students to understand the meaning of songs by providing a visual context for the words. As well, these resources provide variety and diversity to any music program. Teachers are urged to use these resources in their classrooms, taking care to select resources in which illustrations accurately portray the text of the songs and whose content is appropriate for the given students. After children gain familiarity with the resources through listening experiences, these resources offer multiple opportunities for children to engage with music as singers, movers, and instrument players.

Chapter Summary

Even though students with ASD have difficulties with verbal communication (APA, 2013), they are able to perceive and reproduce pitch (Heaton, 2003; Heaton, 2005; Heaton et. al., 1998; Heaton et al., 1999; Simpson & Keen, 2011). Because of this affinity for music, songs and singing are an ideal medium for students on the autism spectrum to experimental vocally and to develop language. From this perspective, songs and singing have the potential to bridge verbal communication through music.

In school settings, vocal communication is not limited to the formation of conventional words joined together to form sentences. Rather, vocal communication is viewed as any verbalizations that are appropriate to the context. This may begin with a student's participation in songs and singing by looking toward the teacher and making laughing-like sounds. As the students continue to practice, their vocal efforts may become discernible words from the students' vocabularies and eventually the words of a given song. This process may unfold over time, perhaps beginning with a student continually repeating one word of a given song and later being able to sing phrases or sections of songs. Eventually, some students acquire a repertoire of songs. In this chapter, materials and strategies related to songs and singing are provided in the hopes that these suggestions will assist teachers to facilitate this work with their students.

Discussion Questions

1. What differences has research established between the ability of students with ASD to perceive, remember, and reproduce pitch (e.g., intervals or melodies) and the abilities of their typically developing peers?
2. How do songs and singing contribute to language acquisition in students with ASD?
3. How do picture books provide opportunities for joint attention among children with ASD and their caregivers?

Notes

1. Thank you to Debbie Stevens for helping with the call and response teaching strategies described here.

2. I express appreciation to Laura Chartrand for suggesting this activity.

4

LISTENING TO MUSIC

TYPICALLY, BABIES BEGIN to cultivate their sense of hearing prior to birth. By the time they are born they are sensitive to the sounds they heard in the womb such as their mother's voice and the language she spoke (Ockelford, 2000). Babies may also be familiar with music they heard before they were born (Ockelford, 2000). Children with learning disabilities may develop their hearing at different rates than their typically developing peers. Nonetheless, they may be able to accurately distinguish sounds, including music.

> It is important, therefore, that children . . . [with disabilities] have access to a rich variety of listening experiences, both within school and beyond, to enable their listening skills to develop as far as possible, and, above all, for the pleasurable sensory and emotional responses that music can engender. (Ockelford, 2000, p. 202)

The ability of children to perceive music depends on their prior experiences with music and their ability to focus on what they hear (Ockelford, 2000). In educational settings, teachers strive to find ways for students to communicate their understanding of music to others (Ockelford, 2000). Communication does not need to rely on spoken words. Rather, children respond to music in many ways. They show their pleasure by smiling and laughing. They indicate their displeasure through physical motions (e.g., by moving away from the source of the sound). They indicate their preferences by pointing to pictures that represent particular musical selections. They demonstrate their understanding of expressive elements through movement (for example, fast music is reflected in fast motions and slow music is reflected in slow motions).

Listening to music requires that children focus their attention on sound, remember what they heard, and respond in ways that are musically appropriate. The ability to listen to music is essential to the development of musical skills (Herrold, 2001). In this chapter, music listening (recorded examples and/or live performances) is discussed as a way for children to focus on and gain an understanding of the music they hear.

Bruscia (1998) outlines five goals for receptive experiences that mirror the outcomes for receptive music listening experiences, described briefly below and explored in this chapter.: to promote receptivity; to stimulate or relax; to foster interpersonal connections; to evoke imagery; and to evoke affective states..

1. To Promote Receptivity: Receptivity is the child's first step toward tolerating music listening experiences. By tolerating these experiences, the child accepts the immediate environment without engaging the fight or flight responses commonly revealed in the behaviors of children on the autism spectrum when faced with anxiety-provoking situations. If a child on the autism spectrum is unable to receive music listening experiences, it is difficult, perhaps impossible, for the child to engage with music and with others in the environment. For this reason, receptivity is the first step towards greater involvement with and through music. Receptivity develops over time as children become accustomed to their environments.

2. To Stimulate or Relax: Recorded music can be an avenue for stimulation or relaxation. A teaching intervention for relaxation and sensory stimulation is described in this chapter along with recommendations for a variety of music that may be used when implementing this strategy.

3. To Foster Interpersonal Connections: Music listening activities provide avenues for children and caregivers to explore joint attention in a calm and relaxed environment. Listening to music supports positive interactions among teachers, caregivers, and children with autism spectrum disorder (ASD), helping these children make social connections within musical environments.

4. To Evoke Imagery: Composers often evoke imagery through their works. In the traditions of Western art music such music is sometimes referred to as program music. For example, in *The Carnival of the Animals*, the composer

Saint-Saëns (1886) portrays the behaviors of numerous animals including lions, chickens, tortoises, and elephants, through music. The extra-musical themes evoked by music provide rich avenues for children to explore objects and events as imagined through music.

5. To Evoke Affective States or Experiences: Music is often thought to express emotions (Ockelford, 2000). For example, it is commonly thought that music written in a major key may be described as *happy* and music written in a minor key may be considered *sad*. Music listening provides avenues for children on the autism spectrum to explore their emotions and to share this understanding with others.

A student's responses to music-based listening experiences are described in text box 4.1.

In teaching music to children on the autism spectrum, the development of receptivity to music and to the planned activities of the music classroom is paramount when helping children connect with others through music. Typically, prior to formal music education, children's aural experiences provide them with a repertoire of familiar sounds (e.g., birds chirping, train whistles, sirens, barking dogs). They may have also obtained some familiarity with music from their home and/or school environments. They may assimilate music from media such as television, radio, and the Internet. As well, caregivers may have used music to promote relaxation and enjoyment or as an avenue for interactions (e.g., using familiar music to support a calm bedtime routine).

TEXT BOX 4.1
CLASSROOM VIGNETTE

Mrs. Lee reflects on how Samuel's responses to music have changed over time. Samuel's first response to music class was to flee. As he was exposed to music he began to show receptivity by looking toward the sound system when he heard recorded music or looking toward the piano when Mrs. Lee played a piece. Music listening as an avenue for relaxation did not have this effect on Samuel until, after several months of exposure, a piece caught his attention. Since that time relaxation sessions have become interactive, as Samuel engages others in nonverbal games (such as peek-a-boo with a scarf). Recently, Samuel used music as a medium for sharing ideas through movement when he pretended to walk through snow while listening to *Snowfall* (Shearing, 1998). He shared his responses to music by choosing icons to indicate whether he thought a piece of music sounded happy or sad.

A first step in assessing a child's receptivity to music is to observe how the child responds to sounds. A child who under-reacts when listening to music may ignore what is heard. In this case, the teacher may direct or re-direct the child's attention using motivational activities or devices such as a stuffed elephant to direct a child's attention to the imagery of the elephant portrayed in *The Carnival of the Animals* (Saint-Saëns, 1886). Knowledge of how the child reacts to music in other contexts assists in the decisions made here. For example, if a child reacts positively when seeing stuffed animals, these props may motivate the child during music listening experiences.

When listening to recorded music, caregivers monitor each student's body language to ascertain whether particular instruments (or groups of instruments) cause discomfort. By observing each student's responses to music (e.g., vocalizations, facial expressions, gestures) teachers learn which children are sensitive to particular stimuli and introduce these sounds into the music classroom sparingly, gradually increasing time spent on particular activities as children become more accustomed to the sounds.

Regardless of whether students over-react or under-react while listening to recorded music, it is recommended that teachers continue to introduce opportunities for students to listen to and interact with music, either through recorded examples or live performances. As music listening becomes a familiar part of the routine, many children begin to focus on the sounds and engage in the planned activities. Teachers and caregivers often continue with music listening experiences even when children are resistant. Persistence is often rewarded.

In this chapter I begin with the identification and review of pedagogical principles for music listening experiences. I then examine ways in which music listening interventions may address challenges for children on the autism spectrum such as joint attention, receptivity, and sensory stimulation I conclude with suggested teaching strategies and musical examples for exploring music's expressive qualities such as dynamics and tempo.

Pedagogical Principles for Listening

Five pedagogical principles for guiding listening experiences are identified in selected music education resources for children in the early grades: musical genres and styles; length; regularity; multisensory engagement; and multiple listening opportunities (Campbell, Scott-Kassner, 2006; Hackett & Lindeman, 2004; Herrold, 2001; Montgomery, 2002). I summarize these below and provide advice for working with children on the autism spectrum.

MUSICAL GENRES AND STYLES

In general, young children are open to listening to a variety of music. For this reason, early years education is an opportune time to expose children to music representing a variety of genres and styles including but not limited to Western art music, jazz, world (cultural) music, new age, and easy listening or popular music.

When choosing recorded music for children on the autism spectrum, educators are advised to pay particular attention to tempo. If children engage in self-stimulating movements, such as rocking or swaying, the music's tempo should be slighter faster than the children's beats (Alvin, 1991). When listening to faster tempi, children are encouraged to adjust their beat to that of the music. This draws their attention from their inside world to the outside environment (Alvin, 1991). As well, children with ASD may be overwhelmed by music featuring a variety of instruments, such as symphonies that use a large number of orchestral instruments, or jazz band arrangements. Teachers may choose to begin listening experiences with music that features a single instrument (e.g., piano). As children gain familiarity and comfort with this music, other selections with variations in instrumentation (tone color) are added to the repertoire.

Students are the teachers' guides in choosing music. Teachers observe the students' body language to see how they react to the music they hear. Their body language and facial expressions indicate whether they enjoy a particular selection and/or the activities that accompany the listening experiences. If a child shows resistance to a particular piece of music, try to motivate his or her attention to the activities or actions of the group. Given the brevity of the selections, the piece is often over before alternate forms of intervention are required (e.g., removing the child from the class). If specific attributes of the recorded music caused the child's frustration, he or she may gain a sense of calm as the group moves to another activity.

Mild discomfort for a particular piece may be due to a number of factors. Perhaps the percussive nature of a piece is overwhelming. A student might place hands over ears to dampen the sound. A student's lack of reception to music may also be due to his or her mind-set on a particular day and may have very little, or nothing, to do with the listening selection or the activities of the class. A classroom vignette about how a child's experiences may influence participation in music class is provided in text box 4.2.

LENGTH

In general, teachers should introduce music listening with short examples (Hackett & Lindeman, 2004; Montgomery, 2002). The length of the selections is expanded gradually as students become increasingly better able to focus on what they hear.

TEXT BOX 4.2
CLASSROOM VIGNETTE

Beverly has had a difficult day. She tripped when she got off the bus. While she was not hurt, the jolt of the fall precipitated a tantrum. The paraprofessional she usually worked with was sick. To top it all off it was pizza day. She really disliked how the food odors permeated the hallways. By the afternoon, Beverly was in no mood to take part in music class. She just wanted to go home.

Hackett and Lindeman suggest that initial listening experiences last between 20 and 30 seconds while Montgomery recommends pieces between 1.5 and 2 minutes in length. The durations for music selections suggested in this chapter range from less than 1 minute to more than 9 minutes depending on the activity that accompanies the listening experience and the children's past experiences in music class.

In my classes, students listen to complete works (or complete sections of works) as much as possible. A particular musical selection may be part of a larger work comprised of numerous items. For example, symphonies may have several movements. In this case, I do not play all movements of the work; however, a selected movement is played in its entirety. Hopefully, through experience, students will learn that a particular activity starts when the music starts and ends when the music ends. In this sense, the end of the music is not the point at which the teacher chooses to stop the music. Rather, it is the point at which the composer concludes the piece. Much, if not most, of the composed music incorporated into music programs in elementary schools ends with a sense of finality on the tonic note of the key in which it is written. With repeated listening, children may learn to discern aurally the feeling of finality portrayed by the sounds and use this information to understand the routines of the class (e.g., when the music finishes, this activity is completed and we move on to the next part of the class).

REGULARLITY

Caregivers may wish to incorporate music into a child's daily routine. In terms of curriculum development and teaching in music, listening to recorded music (or live performance if available), should be integrated into every class. This provides children with opportunities to become familiar with a wide variety of musical styles and genres.

MULTISENSORY ENGAGEMENT

Active listening provides children with opportunities to engage in multi-sensory activities integrating the psychomotor, visual, tactile, and aural senses. In general, children on the autism spectrum are visual learners. If children are listening to music that suggests objects or events outside the music, visual information about the objects or events helps children understand what the music is about. The psychomotor senses are engaged when children are guided to express music through movement. For example, students might listen to the song *Baby Elephant Walk* (Mancini, 1997) while being shown visuals of elephants. They then might move through space creating movements to reflect the baby elephants portrayed in the music.

FAMILIARITY

People tend to like music with which they are familiar. For this reason, students need multiple opportunities to listen to the same selections so the music becomes part of their known repertoire. Teachers monitor their students' progress and use a variety of activities with the same piece of music. This helps children gain familiarity with the selections while avoiding the association of specific activities or routines with specific pieces of music. For example, if students listen to Warlock's (1926) *Pied-en-l'air* every time they dance with scarves, they may adopt a routine of dancing with scarves only when they hear this music. To avoid, or at least reduce, these mindsets students should listen to numerous pieces while dancing through free space, with and without scarves.

Music Listening for Joint Attention, Relaxation, and Sensory Stimulation

Lack of joint attention is a fundamental characteristic of children with ASD (Fein & Dunn, 2007; Jones & Carr, 2004). In joint attention, the child notices something in the environment and, through facial expressions and body language, engages others in what has caught his or her attention. The reward for this action and interaction is that caregivers and children engage in something of common interest. The motivation to initiate joint attention is an important determinant of a child's ability to engage in social endeavors such as playing with other children on the playground (Travis, Sigman, & Ruskin, 2001). Joint attention is central to a child's active involvement in music education events, including activities that involve music listening.

Children on the autism spectrum present challenges for teachers and other caregivers. These children are often resistant to close contact with others. Some children are hypersensitive to physical touch. The establishment of positive relationships relies on helping children develop an acceptance of close proximity to teachers and caregivers (Alvin, 1991). Recorded music provides a relaxing backdrop, creating a positive environment for interpersonal development. The instructional intervention described below nurtures joint attention and allows for gentle sensory stimulation.

INSTRUCTIONAL INTERVENTION: INTERACTION USING SCARVES

Formation: Each child is paired with an adult. They face each other while sitting in chairs or on the floor.

Materials: A selection of multi-colored scarves.

Procedure: The child chooses a brightly colored scarf when provided with two choices and a question such as "Would you like the blue scarf or the yellow scarf?" As they listen to the music, the adult uses a scarf to initiate interaction. The nature of this interaction depends on the child. If the student is sensitive to touch, the adult may begin by holding the scarf in front of the student without making physical contact and then move the scarf away while saying "peekaboo." Over time, the adult begins to touch the student with the scarf. This may begin with a brief touch with the scarf immediately pulled away from the child. As the student becomes accustomed to this sensory stimulation, the adult may begin to slide the scarf along the student's legs or arms.[1] Caregivers may substitute other objects to motivate the child, keeping in mind that whatever object is used should provide a gentle touch. Some experimentation may be needed to discover suitable objects for this activity. Given the success of this intervention when using scarves I rarely sought replacement objects. I did, however, once attempt to substitute large brightly colored feathers (available at craft stores). This was not successful because the children wanted to take the feathers apart and watch the pieces float to the floor.

The extent of a student's involvement in this activity depends on the individual. Nonetheless, interactions represent the following stages of engagement:

- Resist: Resistance is displayed by physical attempts to leave the situation or by verbal indications of displeasure. Teachers and other caregivers need to be persistent. For example, Tommy was an eight-year-old in Mrs. Reinhardt's grade 3 class. He was very sensitive to touch, including being touched by objects and by people. Every time an educational assistant touched him with a scarf he would scream and try to leave the room. One day, Mrs. Reinhardt played a longer piece of music (approximately five minutes in length). Tommy began the activity in his usual manner, crying and squirming in his chair. During the last 30 seconds of the interaction, Tommy's body seemed to relax. He became silent and still. This experience represented a turning point. After he had once settled into the experience, his resistance quickly subsided and, in subsequent classes, he began to engage with his caregiver throughout this activity.

- Ignore: The student may look towards the scarf, but his or her gaze does not follow the object as the adult moves it through space, above the child's head, or towards the child's legs. The student does not provide an outward indication of awareness of the scarf as it touches him or her; nor does the student seem aware of the caregiver when the caregiver attempts to engage the student in the peek-a-boo game.
- Engage: The student looks toward the scarf and watches as it moves through space and gently touches his or her arms or legs. The student may smile or laugh to show approval of the activity. The student may not maintain this interaction throughout the activity, sometimes ignoring the adult and at other times demonstrating engagement.
- Active Involvement: The student looks directly at the adult and/or the scarf throughout most (or all) of the activity. The student's smiles and laughter indicate enjoyment. Through body language the student indicates what motions he or she would like repeated and, through these motions, may show the caregiver what the caregiver should do with the scarf. For example, using hand motions, the student indicates that he or she wants the scarf to wrap around his or her legs. The student actively engages in a game of peek-a-boo.

These descriptions of engagement do not represent a hierarchy through which all students progress. Rather, they represent the types of interactions that may be observed as children with ASD engage (or disengage) during this instructional intervention. A student who is initially resistant to this activity may proceed through all stages of interaction described here. Students on the autism spectrum are sensitive to the world around them and respond to this intervention in different ways depending on their mind set on a particular day. If a student demonstrates behavior at one stage, that does not indicate that he or she has left the previous stage behind. A particular student may respond to this interaction in different ways: for example, actively engaging with the caregiver one week but the next week ignoring the caregiver's encouragements to join in this activity.

SELECTING MUSIC

This intervention lends itself to a variety of music including Western art music, jazz, world (cultural) music, new age, and easy listening or popular music (see tables 4.1 through 4.5 for lists of suggested recorded music with accompanying reference

TABLE 4.1

Western Art Music for Interaction with Scarves

Composer	Artist	Title	Duration	Album	Label	Catalogue Number
Albinoni, T.	The London Virtuoso	Concerto in B flat major, op. 9, no. 11 (movement 2: adagio)	3:26	Albinoni Oboe Concerti	Naxos	8.550739
Bach, J. S.	Nora Shulman; Judy Loman	Siciliano from Sonata no. 2 in E flat major, BWV 1031	2:30	Dance of the Blessed Spirits: Romantic Music for Flute and Harp	Naxos	8.554166
Chopin, F.	Dina Yoffe	Nocturne in F minor op. 55 no. 1	5:16	2 Scherza Nokturny Mazurki	The Fryderyk Chopin Institute	NIFCCD012
Copland, A.	Columbia Symphony Orchestra	Appalachian Spring (Moderato: Coda)	3:25	Copland Conducts Copland	CBS Records Masterworks	MK 42430
Copland, A.	Columbia Symphony Orchestra	Moderato (Like a Prayer)	3:15	Copland Conducts Copland	CBS Records Masterworks	MK 42430
Debussy, C.	Philadelphia Orchestra	Prelude to the Afternoon of a Faun	9:02	Essential Classics	Sony Classical	LSBK53256
Debussy, C.	Philadelphia Orchestra	Nocturnes (no. 1: nuages)	8:19	Essential Classics	Sony Classical	LSBK53256
Elgar	London Philharmonic; Adrian Boult	Serenade for Strings op. 20: Allegretto come prima	3:08	Greensleeves	EMI Laser	CDZ 7 62527 2

Composer	Performer	Title	Duration	Album	Label	Catalog
Handel, G. F.	Concentus Musicus Wien	Concerto Grosso no. 1 in B-dur, op. 3, no. 1 (movement 2: largo)	5:03	Georg Friedrich Handel Concerti Grossi op. 3, numbers 1–6	Teldec	8.35545 ZA
Moreno-Torroba, F.	Paul Madryga	Torija	1:50	Tone Colour Paintbrush	na	HUPM0001
Ravel, M.	Trio Verlaine	Le Tombeau do Couperin	4:04	Fin de siècle: The Music of Debussy and Ravel	Skylark	SKY0801
Vaughan-Williams, R.	London Philharmonic, Adrian Boult	English Folk Song Suite: Intermezzo "My Bonny Boy"	2:52	Greensleeves	EMI Laser	CDZ 7 62527 2
Vivaldi, A.	L'Estro Armonico	Concerto no. 11 in d minor RV565 (largo e spiccato)	2:49	Vivaldi Masterworks	Brilliant Classics	92389/4
Vivaldi, A.	Failoni Chamber Orchestra	Concerto in C major, RV 534, Largo	3:08	Vivaldi Oboe Concerti Vol. 1	Naxos	8.550859
Vivaldi, A.	Failoni Chamber Orchestra	Concerto in C major, RV 450, Larghetto	2:54	Vivaldi Oboe Concerti Vol. 1	Naxos	8.550859
Warlock, P.	Winchester Cathedral Choir and Nicholas Kraemer	Capriol Suite: Pied-en-l'air	2:24	The British Music Collection: Peter Warlock	Decca	000289 470 1992 3
York, A.	Paul Madryga	Waiting for Dawn	3:31	Tone colour paintbrush	na	NUPM0001

TABLE 4.2

Jazz for Interaction with Scarves

Artist	Title	Duration	Album	Label	Catalogue Number
Baker, C.	Somewhere Over the Rainbow	3:28	Somewhere Over the Rainbow	Bluebird	61060-2
Bennett, T.	The Shadow of Your Smile	3:37	The Ultimate Tony Bennett	RPM/COLUMBIA/ Legacy	CK 63570
Benson, G.	C-Smooth	5:27	Standing Together	GRP	GRD 9906
Botti, C.	Night of the Stars	4:42	Night Sessions	Columbia	CK 85753
Brubeck, D.	"Farewell" Jingle Bells	2:59	A Dave Brubeck Christmas	Telarc	CD-83410
Evans, B.	B minor Waltz (for Elaine)	3:12	You Must Believe in Spring	Warner Bros.	3504-2
Evans, B.	You Must Believe in Spring	5:37	You Must Believe in Spring	Warner Bros.	3504-2
Evans, G.	Moon and Sand	4:17	Gil Evans: Jazz Masters 23	Verve	314 521 860-2
Getz, S.	Early Autumn	4:40	The Artistry of Stan Getz: Stan Getz the Best of the Verve Years, vol. 1	Verve	D 225113
Henderson, J.	Dreamer	5:24	Double Rainbow	Verve	314 527 222-2
Herring, V.	Ogrande De Avaio	4:59	Jobim for Lovers	MusicMasters Jazz	01612-65178-2
Peterson, O.	What Child is This	4:47	An Oscar Peterson Christmas	Telarc	CD-83372
Peterson, O.	White Christmas	3:38	An Oscar Peterson Christmas	Telarc	CD-83372
Shearing, G.	In a Calm	3:13	Favorite Things	Telarc Jazz	CD-83398
Shearing, G.	Balulalow	2:17	Christmas with the George Shearing Quintet	Telarc	83438
Shearing, G.	Noel Nouvelet	5:46	Christmas with the George Shearing Quintet	Telarc	83438
Sinatra, F.	Young at Heart	2:50	Capital Years	Capitol	D 297139
Sinclaire, D.	A Peaceful Soul	4:11	Denzal Sinclaire	Verve	4400385782
Sinclaire, D.	I Can See Clearly	4:54	My One and Only Love	Verve	0249884222

TABLE 4.3

Folk Music (and Popular Music in Folk Style) for Interaction with Scarves

Artist	Title	Duration	Album	Label	Catalogue Number
Denver, J.	Falling Leaves	3:35	Take Me Home	Delta Music Group	60354
Joy, G.	Unquiet Grave	3:35	Celtic Secrets	Ancient Echoes	AE104CD
Mitchell, J.	The Circle Game	4:50	Joni Mitchell Hits	Reprise	9 46326-2
Taylor, J.	You've Got a Friend	4:32	James Taylor	Warner Bros.	CD 3113

TABLE 4.4

World Music for Interaction with Scarves

Artist	Title	Duration	Album	Label	Catalogue Number
BecVar, B.	Forever in my Heart	5:12	ARRIBA	Shining Star	SSPCD-119
Chieftains (The)	Tristan and Isolde: Love Theme	2:17	The Chieftains: Film Cuts	RCA Victor	9026-48438-2
Hardiman, R.	Lament	3:23	Michael Flatley's Lord of the Dance	PolyTec	5337572
Maracle, D.	Love Medicine	2:51	Spirit Flutes	Reflections	41318

information). All of the selections included in these tables have been used with this activity to interact with children on the autism spectrum. There is no attempt to weight the relative importance of particular genres by the number of entries. While it is recommended that students have opportunities to listen to a wide variety of music, the emphasis within particular areas is based on the teacher's judgments.

For this activity, listening selections are heard at a relatively quiet volume. In general, the music displays a slow or moderately slow tempo and does not display wide

TABLE 4.5

Easy Listening/Popular Music for Interaction with Scarves

Composer/Artist	Title	Duration	Album	Label	Catalogue Number
Bee Gees	How Can You Mend a Broken Heart?	3:26	One Night Only	Polydor	314 559 220-2
Kenny G.	In the Rain	4:59	Breathless	ARISTA	07822-18646-2
Mancini, H.	Crazy World	4:20	As Time Goes By	RCAVICTOR	BG2 60974
Mancini, H.	Moment to Moment	2:54	The Best of Henry Mancini	BMG Belgium	PA 761/2
McDonald, M.	Tracks of My Tears	3:37	Motown 1	Motown	B000065102
Richie, L.	Say You, Say Me	4:01	Dancing on the Ceiling	Motown	37463 6158-2

variations in dynamics. If the tempo is too fast children do not settle into the activity. This does not imply that children on the autism spectrum do not respond positively to fast tempi. Rather, music with a moderately fast or fast tempo is used for different activities.

The selections listed here range in duration from 2 minutes 10 seconds (Vivaldi's Concerto in D minor [largo]) to 9 minutes and 2 seconds (Debussy's *Prelude to the Afternoon of a Faun*). This activity should be introduced with relatively short selections (approximately 3 minutes in length); longer pieces are introduced when children are familiar with this process. Using music of varying durations assists in meeting the needs of individual children. For example, some children might not settle into this activity until the activity exceeded 5 minutes; other children might be able to maintain their focus for 2 or 3 minutes, but disengage if the duration exceeds this benchmark. When working with individuals, duration is tailored to the predilections of the child, increasing the duration of the music as the child maintains and extends his or her engagement and increases his or her active involvement in the activity.

Children are introduced to a variety of musical styles and instruments in music classes. The examples of Western art music represent a range of orchestrations using instruments from all four families—brass, percussion, strings, and woodwind. Various styles of jazz are represented, including large ensemble (*Manha de Carnival* by Quincy Jones) and solo piano (*In a Calm* by George Shearing). Several solo instruments are featured in small ensembles such as saxophone (Stan Getz) and piano (Oscar Peterson). World music includes native North American flute (David Maracle) and Celtic artists (e.g., The Chieftains). While educators generally want to introduce their students to a variety of music, when beginning this intervention they might choose music with which the children are familiar, gradually increasing their awareness of different styles and genres over time.

The selections listed here are included to assist teachers in choosing appropriate music to use with their students. Much, if not most, of this music is available online. In terms of Western art music, several versions of the same composed pieces may be available. Given that in this genre of music musicians are generally charged with reproducing music as the composers intend, slight differences in rendition will probably not interfere with the outcomes of instruction. In fact, these differences may reinforce the idea of personal interpretation of Western art music. Conversely, in the jazz idiom, the performers' intent is to create something of their own from the blue print created by the composer. For this reason, readers may wish to choose performances by the artists listed (or similar performances by alternate artists) for use in the educational intervention described here. While many alternate versions of the same piece may be appropriate for use with this activity, teachers should preview the music before using it in their classrooms to ensure that the instrumentation and tempo of the music provides a suitable accompaniment for this activity. For readers interested in adding to their personal collections of music, the recording *Songs from the Secret Garden* (Secret Garden, 1995) is an ideal resource as every one of the tracks provides an appropriate accompaniment for this activity.

Teachers observe their students' behaviors as, through their body language and verbalizations, children inform caregivers of their preferences for particular music. As we listen to our students we learn how to involve them in the selection of music. For example, Chet Baker's rendition of *Somewhere Over the Rainbow* was brought to class based on a child's repeated requests for trumpet. Teachers are encouraged to experiment with their own selections, observing the children's reactions to assess the suitability of their choices.

Tempo and Dynamics

Two common elements in music are tempo and dynamics. *Tempo* is the speed of the underlying pulse or beat. *Dynamics* refers to the intensity or volume of sounds (Gardstrom, 2007). While it is possible to denote individual selections as loud or quiet and fast or slow, identification of tempo and dynamics is often comparative, not absolute.

DYNAMICS

Music listening experiences provide students with ASD opportunities to refine their aural discrimination by listening to music and identifying whether it is loud or quiet. The ease with which children discriminate levels of dynamics depends on the characteristics of the music. Sometimes music is obviously loud or quiet. Other times students need to listen to two pieces, one loud and one relatively quiet, and make this determination through comparisons. Suggested examples for music listening are provided in Table 4.6. Estimations of dynamics are determined through personal judgments of dynamics in music. Readers are encouraged to experiment with additional examples, taking into account their own perceptions of dynamics and tempo and the musical preferences and perspectives of their students.

When choosing listening examples to contrast quiet and loud, it is important to vary the tempo of the music. While it is appropriate to listen to some quiet music that is slow and some loud music that is fast, doing so consistently may lead students to assume that this generalization holds true for all music. For this reason, students also need the opportunity to listen to quiet music that is fast and loud music that is

TABLE 4.6

Dynamics and Tempo

Composer	Title	Duration	Album	Label	Catalogue Number	Dynamics	Tempo
Grieg, E.	In the Hall of the Mountain King	2:11	Sir John Barbirolli	Memoir Classics	446	Gradually getting louder (*crescendo*)	Gradually getting faster (*accelerando*)
Haydn, J.	Symphony No. 94 in G major (movement II: andante)	6:35	Haydn London Symphonies (vol. 2—Nos. 94, 101 & 102)	CHANDOS early music	CHAN 0662	Various	Andante
Ravel, M.	Valses nobles et sentimentales (movement 1: Modere)	1:23	Ravel	Sony Essential Classics	LSBK 48163	Loud	Medium fast
Rossini, G.	William Tell Overture (final section)	3:19	Rossini 7 overtures	London	400 049 - 2	Loud	Fast
Saint-Saëns, C.	Kangaroos	1:00	Camille Saint-Saëns	Excelsior	EXL-2-4290	Quiet	Moderately slow
Saint-Saëns, C.	Wild Asses	:35	Camille Saint-Saëns	Excelsior	EXL-2-4290	Loud	Moderately slow
Satie, E.	Danses de travers II	1:25	*Piano works:* Gymnopedies & Gnossiennes	Philips Classics	4681602	Quiet	Medium fast

(*continued*)

TABLE 4.6

Continued

Composer	Title	Duration	Album	Label	Catalogue Number	Dynamics	Tempo
Mussgorsky, M.	Battle of the Unhatched Chicks	1:12	Pictures at an Exhibition	Deutsche Grammophon	410 033-2	Quiet with long accented note and *crescendo* toward the end of the piece	Fast
Warlock, P.	Capriol Suite: Pavane	2:08	The British Music Collection: Peter Warlock	Decca	000289 470 1992 3	Quiet	Slow
Warlock, P.	Capriol Suite: Basse-danse	1:40	The British Music Collection: Peter Warlock	Decca	000289 470 1992 3	Loud	Fast
Warlock, P.	Capriol Suite: Bransles	1:58	The British Music Collection: Peter Warlock	Decca	000289 470 1992 3	Quiet	Fast
Warlock, P.	Capriol Suite: Tordion	1:06	The British Music Collection: Peter Warlock	Decca	000289 470 1992 3	Gradually getting quieter (*decrescendo*)	Moderate
Rimsey-Korsakov, N.	Flight of the Bumble Bee	1:02	Greatest Hits: The Canadian Brass	RCA	1-4733	Quiet-loud-quiet	Fast

slow so they judge the dynamic quality on the volume on the music without relying on assumptions about tempo when making these decisions. This need for variety is accounted for in the selections listed in Table 4.6.

Individuals with ASD often have difficulties focusing on a single element in their environment. Every detail is important to them and they try to attend to everything. It is possible that this tendency transfers to music listening. In such cases, identifying the dynamics of music may be a challenging task. To assist these students, teachers might begin focusing on dynamics with "Kangaroos" (quiet) and "Wild Asses" (loud) from Saint-Saëns' (1886) *The Carnival of the Animals*. Since both of these pieces have a similar tempo, students might be better able to focus on dynamics without their attention being interrupted by judgments of tempo. After students are able to identify loud and quiet in these two selections, teachers might contrast the loud "Wild Asses" to one of the quiet pieces listed in Table 4.6, such as Warlock's *Pavane*. Warlock's compositions *Pavane* and *Bransle* could then be used to provide a contrast between music that is quiet and slow and quiet and fast.

After students are able to discriminate loud and quiet, they may be ready to distinguish more refined changes in dynamics such as music that gradually becomes louder (*crescendo*) and music that gradually becomes quieter (*decrescendo*). These phenomena are represented by Grieg's *In the Hall of the Mountain King* (*crescendo*) and Warlock's *Tordion* (*decrescendo*). Teachers must remain aware that children on the autism spectrum may be particularly sensitive to dynamic contrasts, especially if these contracts occur unexpectedly. For example, in Haydn's Symphony no. 94 in G Major commonly referred to as the *Surprise Symphony*, children may be disturbed by the *surprise* (an accented chord within the main theme of the third movement). Given the length of this movement (6:35), teachers may want to play only the first section of the third movement so that students have an opportunity to hear the accented chord played towards the conclusion of the first statement of the main theme.

It is important that teachers take care with the terminology used to describe dynamics in music. For example, dynamics are often described as *loud* and *soft*. Children may confuse these expressions of dynamics in music with the words *hard* and *soft* used to describe textures (e.g., the floor is hard and the carpet is soft). Given this, it is important that children be given multiple opportunities to hear music and identify these dynamic levels to gain an understanding of how the words *quiet* and *loud* are used to describe music.

Teachers may also consider when to introduce the Italian words for dynamics as this is the terminology commonly used in music. If working in an inclusive setting, the teacher may choose to introduce the words *loud* and *quiet* followed shortly by the Italian terms used by musicians (*forte* and *piano*, respectively). When doing so, it is important for the teacher and/or instructional assistants help children with special needs by emphasizing the English words if children have difficulty interpreting the Italian terms. If working only with children with limited verbal abilities, educators may choose to limit instruction to the English descriptors.

Teaching strategies
Loud or quiet

DIRECT INSTRUCTION. Students listen to selected loud music while the instructor points to a picture, say, of a crow with the word *loud* printed underneath it, Students then listen to quiet music while the instructor points to picture, say, of a mouse with the word *quiet* printed underneath it. These animals are suggested representations of loud and quiet. Individual teachers choose objects to represent quiet and loud in ways that are appropriate for their students' environments. No specific order is intended in this description. Teachers may begin with either quiet or loud, provided that students have the opportunity to hear contrasting examples representing both levels of dynamics. This activity is repeated across several lessons until students gain an understanding of how the concepts of loud and quiet relate to music. Depending on the background of particular students, the words *quiet* and *loud* could be substituted for the pictures.

GUIDED INSTRUCTION. Children are shown two cards. As indicated in the previous activity, one card illustrates quiet and the other illustrates loud. Children listen to the music and indicate which illustration best reflects what they hear. Depending on the background experience of the students and the particular music, students may need to listen to both pieces before making this judgment.

Getting louder (crescendo)/*getting quieter* (decrescendo)

After children understand loud and quiet, they may be introduced to music in which the dynamics gradually change from quiet to loud (*crescendo*) or from loud to quiet (*decrescendo*).

DIRECT INSTRUCTION. Students listen to selected music while the instructor points to a visual of the crescendo symbol used in music with the words *gradually getting louder* written underneath it. Students listen to music while the instructor points to a visual of the decrescendo symbol used in music with the words *gradually getting quieter* written underneath it. No specific order is intended in this description. Teachers may begin with either *crescendo* or *decrescendo*. This activity is repeated across several lessons until students gain an understanding of how the concept of *crescendo* and *decrescendo* relate to dynamics in music.

GUIDED INSTRUCTION. Children are shown two cards: one illustrates crescendo and the other illustrates decrescendo, as indicated in the previous example. Children listen to a piece of music and indicate which illustration best reflects what they hear.

TEMPO

The ease with which students discriminate tempo depends on the characteristics of the specific music. Sometimes music is obviously fast or slow. Sometimes it is difficult to decide whether a piece is fast or slow without a means of comparison. Suggested examples for music listening are provided in Table 4.6. Estimations of tempo are not absolute. I have provided options of music that is fast and slow that include both loud and quiet levels of dynamics, but the designations are based on my estimations. Readers are encouraged to experiment with additional examples, taking into account their own perceptions of dynamics and tempo and the musical preferences and perceptions of their students.

When choosing listening examples to contrast slow and fast, it is important to vary the dynamics of the music. While it is appropriate to listen to some slow music that is quiet and some fast music that is loud, doing so consistently may lead students to assume that this generalization holds true for all music. For this reason, students also need opportunities to listen to slow music that is loud and fast music that is quiet so they judge the tempo based on what they hear rather than on assumptions about dynamics when making these decisions. This need for variety is accounted for in the selections listed in Table 4.6. Two of Warlock's compositions, *Pavane* and *Bransle* provide a contrast in tempo with the first piece slow and the second one faster. Both pieces are quiet, allowing students to concentrate on comparing tempi without being confused by changes in dynamics. After students are able to identify tempo in these pieces, others with a contrast in dynamics, such as Offenbach's *Infernal Gallop* or the final section of Rossini's *William Tell Overture* could be added. Both of these pieces are fast and loud.

Teachers may also consider when to introduce the Italian words for tempo as this is the terminology often used in the discipline of music. If working in an inclusive setting, the teacher may introduce the words *slow* and *fast* followed shortly by the Italian terms used by musicians such as *adagio* (slow and stately) and *allegro* (fast, cheerful). When doing so, it is important for the teacher and/or instructional assistants to help children with special needs by emphasizing the English words if children have difficulty interpreting the Italian terms. If working with children with limited verbal abilities, educators may choose to limit instruction to the English descriptors.

After children are able to discriminate fast and slow, they may be able to distinguish more refined changes in tempo such as music that gradually becomes faster (*accelerando*). For example, Grieg's *In the Hall of the Mountain King* begins quietly and slowly. As the theme repeats, the music becomes faster and louder. Thus, in one piece listeners hear both a *crescendo* and an *accelerando*.

As students refine their aural awareness, they may be able to judge finer distinctions in tempo including *grave* (slow and solemn) and *presto* (very fast). Teaching strategies described here are limited to suggestions for teaching fast and slow as well as getting faster. Individual educators may adapt these strategies to teach finer discriminations of tempo.

Teaching strategies
Fast and slow
DIRECT INSTRUCTION. Students listen to fast music while the instructor points to a picture of, say, a rabbit with the word *fast* printed underneath it (if written language is appropriate for students). Students listen to slow music while the instructor points to a picture of, say, a turtle with the word *slow* printed underneath it. No specific order is intended in this description. Students may begin by listening to music that is either fast or slow, provided that they have the opportunity to hear contrasting examples representative of these tempi in order to compare one to the other. This activity is repeated across several lessons until students gain an understanding of how the concepts of fast and slow relate to music. The illustrations are modified to correspond with the level of the students so that, when appropriate, they are shown the printed words without the accompanying pictures.

GUIDED INSTRUCTION. Children are shown two cards: one illustrates slow and the other illustrates fast. Children listen to a piece of music and indicate which illustration best reflects what they hear. Depending on the background experience of the students, teachers may begin this activity by asking them to listen to two examples, one fast and one slow. As they gain experience teachers may gauge the students' aural discrimination by asking them to indicate whether a piece is fast or slow without comparing two pieces. After children understand fast and slow, they may be introduced to music in which the tempo gradually changes from slow to fast.

Gradually getting faster (accelerando)
DIRECT INSTRUCTION. Students listen to selected music while the instructor points to the phrase *gradually getting faster*. The procedure is repeated across several lessons until students gain an understanding of this concept in music.

GUIDED INSTRUCTION. Students listen to a selected piece of music. They are presented with three cards that indicate three different descriptions of tempo: fast, slow, and gradually getting faster. Students choose the card that best describes what they hear.

Chapter Summary

Children on the autism spectrum are capable of responding positively to a wide variety of music listening experiences. In this chapter, listening to music is explored as a vehicle for relaxation and sensory stimulation and as a means for gaining joint attention between children with ASD and their caregivers. Listening increases understanding when children are provided direct and guided instruction to discern expression in music through dynamics and tempo. Most of the activities presented in this chapter require that students passively receive music and make judgments based on what they hear. More active engagements are not generally achieved through listening alone but, rather, when listening to music is combined with other forms of engagement. For this reason, listening to music is revisited in the following two chapters with activities that combine music listening with moving (Chapter 5) and playing instruments (Chapter 6).

Discussion Questions

1. How do listening experiences contribute to a balanced music program for students with ASD?
2. What music from your own collection might be suited to the educational strategies described in this chapter?
3. What possibilities do you see for using the activities described in this chapter with your students?

Note

1. The author expresses appreciation to Shannon Vogel who suggested this technique.

5

....

MOVING

TEACHERS OFTEN OBSERVE that children on the autism spectrum move their bodies in ways that differ from children who do not have autism. Some children with autism spectrum disorder (ASD) rock back and forth to their own beat; some children run in free space with no apparent goals for their actions. Other students may sit on the floor and spin in circles. Challenges in successfully completing psychomotor tasks have significant implications for how individuals with ASD perform day-to-day tasks such as getting dressed, eating, and brushing their teeth (Hilton, Zhand, White, Klohr, & Constantive, 2011). Researchers estimate that between 80% and 90% of individuals with ASD demonstrate non-typical motor behaviors (Hilton et al., 2011). Therefore, it would seem that general motor deficiencies are an essential characteristic of autism.

Children on the autism spectrum generally display poor movement skills in comparison to their typically developing peers (Staples & Reid, 2010). This is evident early in their development, beginning with challenges in the movements needed to crawl or walk as toddlers (Dziuk et al., 2007). As children get older they experience difficulties with basic motor control such as with coordinating the left and right sides of their bodies. They also experience difficulties performing basic locomotor skills such as walking or hopping and rudimentary psychomotor skills such as throwing or catching a ball (Rinehart, Bradshaw, Brereton, & Tonge, 2001).

Slow or uncoordinated movements in the upper body, specifically the head and arms, may limit the effectiveness with which children on the autism spectrum are able to reach, point, give, and show (Bhat, Landa, & Galloway, 2011). These are all important components in initiating and maintaining joint attention with others. Individuals who experience difficulties with fundamental motor skills tend to avoid social play, are not asked to play with others, and have fewer friends than their typically developing peers. These difficulties with motor skill development restricts their engagements in sports and other recreational activities and can lead to isolation as children with ASD retreat from social interactions with others.

Music acts as an "auditory frame of reference for movement" (Ockelford, 2000, p. 204). Engagement through music has the potential to bridge the gap between children on the autism spectrum and other individuals in their environments (e.g., parents, siblings, teachers, peers). As children respond to music and music making they interact with others in ways that facilitate the development of practical movement skills. This provides children with ASD multiple opportunities to practice and improve motor proficiency, as illustrated in text box 5.1

This chapter begins with an overview of selected research literature that profiles the challenges encountered by children with ASD in relation to motor development including:

- Gait and Coordination
- Motor Planning
- Object Control
- Imitation

Findings from this literature guide the structure and content of the teaching strategies that follow.

TEXT BOX 5.1
CLASSROOM VIGNETTE

Alexander does not like recess. He never plays tag with the other students. He does not know the rules for the game and thinks that he would not be any good at it anyway. He often stumbles when he runs and would not like to be caught or tagged by another student. He sits by himself and watches the clouds roll by. Music class is better than recess. The teacher explains the rules for the games and the beats she plays on the drum help him to move his feet at the right time when the students walk around the room.

Motor Development

GAIT AND COORDINATION

The ability to move one's body through space (locomotion) depends on the ability to maintain equilibrium throughout the body. The initial development of this control is the head-straightening reflex that allows an individual to keep the head erect while the body is inclined (Vernazza-Martin et al., 2005). Second is adjustment to the pelvic region that stabilizes and supports the upper body during movements in the feet.

Individuals on the autism spectrum generally display differences in how they move their bodies through space when compared to peers who exhibit typical patterns of development. The gait of individuals with autism is typified by a slower pace and smaller strides. As well, walking patterns in individuals on the autism spectrum sometimes lack the typical heel-toe pattern and display less movement in the arms than is exhibited in typical development (Bhat et al., 2011). Individuals with ASD also display less range of motion in their ankles and less flexing in their knees than their typically developing peers (Hallett et al., 1993). When walking through free space, children with ASD are generally less able to modify gait patterns in response to feedback from the immediate environment (Lagasse & Hardy, 2013). Thus, these individuals may have difficulty maneuvering around the objects (desks, chairs, bookcases, cupboards, learning centers) found in typical classroom environments.

An examination of gait (or locomotion) in individuals with ASD illustrates possible coordination challenges experienced by these children. Morin and Reid (1985) observed that children on the autism spectrum experienced difficulties in coordinating arm movements in running tasks. In more recent research, Staples and Reid (2010) found that individuals with ASD had difficulty coordinating the two sides of their bodies for tasks that required the use of both arms and legs.

MOTOR PLANNING

Motor planning is an essential component in advanced motor skills (Hardy & LaGasse, 2013). It relies on several processes including the initiation of an act and the coordination of separate elements into a sequence that allows the individual to achieve a particular goal (Todd, 2012). Typically, children are able to execute motor plans by the age of seven (Todd, 2012). In contrast, individuals with ASD have difficulty combining separate actions into a single response; rather, they view each part of the sequence as a single, independent act (Hardy & LaGasse, 2013). Difficulties with motor planning are one of the earliest signs of autism and may be at the root of commonly held descriptions of persons with ASD as "clumsy" (Rinehart et al.,

2001; Schmitz, Martineau, Barthélémy, & Assaiante, 2003). Children who have problems with motor planning continue to experience difficulties throughout their lives (Todd, 2012). These individuals often understand what movements they are expected to perform, but have problems performing movement sequences correctly. These children may be able to perform single movements in isolation, but experience difficulties when asked to perform a sequence of movements. For example, in a music class, a child may be able to complete rowing motions while singing the song *Row, Row, Row Your Boat* but may experience difficulties in performing the motions for the song *The Eency Weency Spider* (a traditional song also known as *The Itsy Bitsy Spider*) as this requires the child to sequence movements (see Table 5.1). Difficulty with performing sequences is illustrated in text box 5.2.

TABLE 5.1

The Eency Weency Spider Lyrics	Movement Sequence
The eency weency spider went up the water spout.	Touch the tip of the thumb on one hand to the tip of the forefinger of the other hand. Alternate this position from hand to hand to represent the spider walking up the spout.
Down came the rain and washed the spider out.	Move arms in higher to lower motion to illustrate the rain washing the spider out of the spout.
Out came the sun and dried up all the rain.	Raise hands and arms above the head toward the sun.
And the eency weency spider went up the spout again.	Repeat the first movement.

TEXT BOX 5.2
CLASSROOM VIGNETTE

Tom has problems completing tasks that require him to sequence several movements. Students in Mr. Abbott's class play a game in which they sit in a circle and pass a ball from one student to the next at the same tempo at which the teacher improvises at the piano. This requires that Tom stabilize his posture while sitting on the floor, hold the ball in his left hand when it is passed to him by another student, transfer the ball to the right hand, and pass the ball to the next student. All of this must be done with sufficient force to pass the ball, but with not so much force that the ball rolls across the room or to the middle of the circle.

OBJECT CONTROL

Object control is a skill that is routinely used in day-to-day activities. For example, children are expected to reach and grasp utensils (forks, knives, and spoons) for eating; they grasp toothbrushes for cleaning their teeth and combs for untangling their hair. In music class, children hold musical instruments. They grasp a variety of props (e.g., streamers or scarves) to take part in interactive activities.

Sumway-Cook and Woollacott (2007) describe the requirements to develop reaching, grasping, and manipulating skills. These requirements are summarized below, followed by description of their application to music education:

- Locating a visual target; requires the coordination of eye-head movements
- Reaching, involving the movement of the arm and hand in space as well as balance and correct posture
- Grasping, including grip formation, grasp, and release
- Manipulating, entailing the appropriate use of tools and/or objects

For example:

- A drum is placed on a table. The teacher points to the drum, while saying "play drum." The student turns his or her head toward the drum.
- The student walks to the table, leans his or her upper body over the table, and reaches out arms and hands to the drum.
- The student grasps the drum by the handle on its underside and carries the drum back to his or her chair.
- The student holds the drum by the handle with one hand and plays the drum with the palm of the free hand.

The reach-to-grasp response relies on "muscle tone, muscle strength, and coordination" (Sumway-Cook & Woollacott, 2007, p. 455) including the use of muscles to support the upper body and head during reaching and the use of muscles in the shoulder, elbow, and wrist in the forward motion of the arm. The postural requirements vary in relation to the task. For example, it is easier for a child to reach and grasp a musical instrument while in a seated position than if the child is standing as the latter position requires the child to stabilize the legs and body. When the processes involved in reaching and grasping are analyzed as separate components one sees that even relatively simple tasks, such as preparing to play a percussion instrument, require multiple processes such as planning and following through to task completion. Typically developing children make improvements in these areas between the ages of 2 and 4. Children on the autism spectrum often exhibit delays in these behaviors (Hughes, 1996). The difficulties are attributed to their inability to plan and execute tasks that require a series of actions (Mari et al., 2003). In addition, Sumway-Cook and Woollacott (2007) note that the visual processing required to complete these tasks is more complex when the person is expected to reach across the vertical midline of the body. As a result, arm movements completed on the same side of the body (the right arm reaching to the right side), called ipsilateral movements, are completed more quickly and more accurately than movements that require an individual to reach across the body (right arm reaching to the left side), called contralateral movements.

IMITATION

Scott (2016) provides a more extensive examination of how children with ASD learn through imitation in general and, more specifically, how they learn about music through imitation. During early development, young children typically acquire new skills by imitating others during interactive play. Children with ASD demonstrate delays in the ability to imitate others early in life (Smith & Bryson, 2007). Challenges in performing tasks that require imitation remain as these children become adults (Bhat et al., 2011). Difficulties in motor imitation do not indicate that children on the autism spectrum are not able to imitate another's actions (Williams, Whiten, & Singh, 2004). Rather, children on the autism spectrum imitate actions less often and with less accuracy than their typically developing peers (Williams et al., 2004). It is possible that individuals with autism are not motivated to imitate others (Hobson & Lee, 1999). This lack of motivation limits the opportunities they have to practice and refine these skills (Rogers, Bennetto, McEvoy, & Pennington, 1996).

In describing how children with ASD respond to motor imitation, Smith and Bryson (2007) identified two types of gestures:

- *Meaningful gestures* are upper body movements that have a social and/or cultural intent such as waving hello or goodbye (see Figure 5.1, left frame). The completion of a meaningful gesture requires that the children understand and remember the meaning associated with the gesture and are able to enact the visual and motor processes required to complete the movement
- *Nonmeaningful gestures* are movements that do not have a clearly defined social and/or cultural meaning, such as placing one's hand on one's head (see Figure 5.1, right frame). The completion of nonmeaningful gestures does not rely on remembering and/or understanding previous experiences.

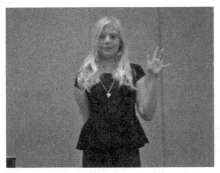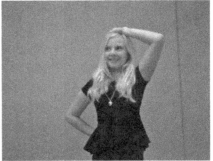

FIGURE 5.1 Meaningful (left) and Nonmeaningful (right) Gestures

The imitator only needs to be able to visually perceive the motion and implement the motor actions needed to imitate the gesture.

Children on the autism spectrum find it easier to perform meaningful than nonmeaningful gestures (Vanvuchelen, Roeyers, & De Weert, 2007). These researchers concluded that the difficulties children on the autism spectrum experience in completing gestures are due to challenges in perceiving the visual and motor components of the tasks (Smith & Bryson, 2007; Vanvuchelen et al., 2007). As well, Ingersoll and Schreibman (2006) observed that children on the autism spectrum do not communicate through gesture as often as their typically developing peers. This limits their opportunities to practice and refine this skill.

Educational Experiences Integrating Movement and Music

Children with ASD often know what movements they want to complete, but have difficulties performing the required motions. Consequently, there is a need for instructional interventions that help children on the spectrum to better manage their movements. The change of behaviors that emerges from these interventions has the potential to improve how these children interact within their physical environments, including communications between children on the spectrum and their typically developing peers.

Campbell and Scott-Kassner (2006) claim that movement is foundational to how children learn through play:

From early childhood, children move playfully as they sing songs associated with games, actions, and dances. The melodies of action songs and singing games draw from children the movements they have naturally encountered in their free play. These movements are recalled and organized by children to express the song's rhythmic and expressive qualities. (p. 123)

Activities incorporating music and movement create learning environments well suited to the educational needs of children with ASD. The foundational properties of movement (e.g., energy, force, space, speed, and weight) are addressed systematically through instruction, with these properties modeled by teachers, instructional assistants, and peers. Integrated activities using music and movement create environments in which children are able to take risks as, through continued practice, they gain facility in coordinating their physical movements with music.

FEATURES OF MOVEMENT INTERVENTIONS

In this section several features of movement interventions for children on the autism spectrum are explored, including:

- Body awareness
- Spatial awareness
- Understanding of movement and acquisition of a movement vocabulary
- Effort and energy (force, speed, and weight) in movement
- Object control
- Opportunities for practice
- Freedom to experiment through movement
- Collaboration

Body awareness

Body awareness relates to the individual's understanding of posture. It also relates to the individual's understanding of the relationships among the various parts of the body, and how these parts move in place (nonlocomotor movement) and space (locomotor movement). Landy and Burridge (1999) identify seven elements necessary for achieving and maintaining proper posture. Each is described below.

- Balance: Posture begins with a sense of balance, which is the foundation from which all movements emerge. Balance may be an obvious component in movements that require students to stand and/or move through space. It is also important for sitting activities as it is the sense of balance that allows the individual to maintain an upright body position. A narrow stance (commonly referred to as the distance between the feet) and unnecessary upper body movements are common causes of poor balance for individuals in standing positions.

- Head Stability: The head is the reference from which the other parts of the body move. Eye-to-object focus, body position, and balance are all affected negatively if a child is unable to control the movements of the head.
- Body Alignment: Writing from the perspective of physical education, Landy and Burridge (1999) describe the role of posture in motor activities in which the body is aligned to a target (e.g., a golf ball) or in which body alignment contributes to moving an object forward in a straight line (e.g., a baseball). In these cases, body alignment contributes to the force and accuracy of the movements. In music, body alignment contributes to the facility with which one plays non-pitched percussion instruments.
- Flexed Knees: When standing, knees should be slightly flexed. Flexed knees contribute to stable balance and allow for shifts in balance from one leg to the other. Flexed knees also help to cushion locomotor movements such as walking or hopping. When knees are flexed, individuals experience less fatigue in the legs.
- Body Height Consistency: Many movements (e.g., running, walking) require that the height of the body remains consistent. If children continually bend or straighten their bodies they may have difficulties maintaining their balance.
- Transfer of Weight and Force: The transfer of weight is necessary to achieve efficiency and force in movement. Locomotor activities in music classrooms (e.g., stepping the beat and/or subdivisions of the beat) rely on the weight on the back leg being transferred to the front leg as the body is propelled forward.
- Focused eyes: When balancing, eyes should be focused on a fixed point. When manipulating objects, eyes need to be focused on the target for the activity (e.g., when playing the hand drum, eyes are focused on the hand as it strikes the instrument).

Body awareness requires that children understand how the different parts of the body move. For example:

- Parts of the body may be active while others are inactive (e.g., the upper body moves while the legs are still).
- Parts of the body are related to each other in terms of sidedness (e.g., the right arm or the left arm).

- Parts of the body may move in unison (e.g., both hands clap together) (Buschner, 1994).
- Parts of the body may move in opposition (e.g., the right arm stretches upward and the left arm stretches downward).

Relevant educational interventions are explored later in this chapter in the sections on nonlocomotor and locomotor movement.

Spatial awareness

In music classes, children must adapt to two perspectives of space—personal space and general space. Personal space is the space within immediate reach of the child while sitting in a desk or chair, sitting on the floor, or standing. General space is the area defined by the walls of the classroom. Increasing spatial awareness requires that children have opportunities to explore movement within their personal spaces (nonlocomotor movement) and movement that requires them to propel their bodies through space (locomotor movement). Locomotor movement also requires that students negotiate their bodies around other people and objects in the room (Buschner, 1994), thus increasing the difficulty of movement activities. For this reason, children need numerous opportunities to control their movements in personal space before moving through general space (Buschner, 1994).

Children on the autism spectrum have difficulties perceiving the boundaries of personal space. If children are sitting on chairs or in desks, these objects provide visual markers for this concept. If children are sitting on the floor in an open space, they may need a visual marker such as individual squares of carpet to delineate the space. Rather than distinguishing students with ASD from their peers, all students may be asked to sit on squares of carpet. These visual markers aid classroom management. For example, after children travel through space pretending to fly like birds, they might all follow the teacher's request to go back to their places (e.g., squares of carpet). Whole class procedures such as these create a welcoming and inclusive environment as students with ASD are not distinguished from their peers. Classroom activities that help children to understand personal space are explored in text box 5.3.

Awareness of energy or effort

Energy or effort describes the force (weight), tempo (time), or flow of movements. Elements of energy or effort relevant to the movement activities described in this chapter are summarized in Table 5.2. Feierabend and Kahan (2003) is recommended to readers interested in learning more about energy and effort in movement.

TEXT BOX 5.3
CLASSROOM VIGNETTE

Mrs. Carter wants students in kindergarten to understand the relation of their bodies in space. Music instruction begins with activities in which children explore personal space. The students sit on individual squares of carpet and reach their arms in all directions around this space. Students then explore the general space in the room. They play a game in which they walk around the room and freeze when the music stops.

TABLE 5.2

Energy or Effort	
Energy or Effort	Movement
FORCE (WEIGHT)	
light	free and flowing, muscles relaxed
heavy	weighty, relatively slow, muscles somewhat tense
gentle	calm, soft, light, soothing, restful
strong	physically powerful, sturdy
TEMPO (TIME)	
fast	quick, rapid
slow	long, drawn-out, leisurely
FLOW	
smooth	even, level
jagged	uneven, choppy, rough
tense	stiff, tight muscles
relaxed	calm, peaceful

Movement vocabulary

Related to spatial awareness, children need to understand the vocabulary used to describe physical movements. Movement vocabulary common to music classes is described in Table 5.3.

Object control

In music class, movement activities are combined with reach-to-grasp and object control. The reach-to-grasp motion comes into play when children hold musical instruments or props such as balls, scarves, streamers, or hula hoops. Children

TABLE 5.3

Movement Vocabulary

Non-locomotor (in place)	Locomotor (through space)	Force/effort
straight/curved	backward/forward	big/small
in front/behind	straight/sideways	slow/fast
next to/across from	clockwise/counterclockwise	heavy/light
right/left	right/left	strong/weak
over/under	diagonal	
face-to-face/back-to-back	zigzag	
stretch/bend	over/under	
shake/shrug/swing	slide/glide	
turn	walk/hop/gallop/skip	

reach-to-grasp objects from a seated position when items are handed to them. They reach to grasp from a standing position when requested to walk to a place in the room where these objects are stored, choose the required object, and return to their personal space. Object control is needed to play musical instruments appropriately and to handle the props as suited to the given tasks.

Practice

Many children on the autism spectrum seem to lack an innate sense of coordination. Their movements appear awkward or out-of-sync with those of the rest of the class. These children need multiple opportunities to practice and refine movements by engaging in numerous challenging and enjoyable activities. With time, effort, and patience children with ASD can improve their ability to control their whole bodies and parts of their bodies as they move in place and through space, increasingly refining their movements over time.

Creativity

Through taking part in structured movement activities in which the leader directs the activities (e.g., everyone crouches on the ground and moves upwards to reach the sky), children gain a repertoire of body movements. Less structured activities allow the students to apply their understanding and skills in movement to communicate in creative ways. For example, they might use smooth, gentle, and slow movements to express a sunny day and jagged, forceful, and fast movements to represent a storm. Teachers guide these ideas by supplying an impetus for movement such as familiar objects from nature (e.g., trees or flowers), insects (bumble bees, lady bugs), or animals (bears, elephants, dogs, cats). The children's memories and imaginations come into play as they create their own movements to represent their thoughts. Children's responses are limited to their personal frames of reference. For example, the teacher's request that students move like bears in the forest assumes that students are familiar with bears. They also need to know what is meant by the word *forest*. Teachers may supplement verbal directions with concrete information (e.g., objects or photographs) to help children with ASD relate what the teacher is saying to their previous knowledge.

Collaboration

Music-based activities provide children with opportunities to collaborate with others while they acquire facility with movement through music-based activities. Children with ASD are members of an ensemble when they join group music-making activities such as singing songs while performing the requisite actions or playing rhythm instruments to accompany these songs. They interact with partners when they imitate a partner's motions using rhythm sticks (see Chapter 6, Playing Instruments). They become aware of others as they manage their movements within their own space and through the free space shared with others.

GENERAL GUIDELINES FOR TEACHING MOVEMENT

The following guidelines for teaching are relevant regardless of the specifics of the movement activity in which the children are involved. These guidelines are applicable to working with all students; specifications for working with children on the autism spectrum are noted.

- If possible, arrange for an open space that allows plenty of room for both nonlocomotor and locomotor movement (Hackett & Lindeman, 2004; Montgomery, 2002).
- Incorporate movement activities into every lesson (Montgomery, 2002).
- Suit movement activities to the skill levels of the students, keeping in mind that it may take longer for children on the autism spectrum to master these activities than their typically developing peers.
- Begin with activities using large muscle movements (Anderson & Lawrence, 2010).
- The tempo for classroom movement activities should be faster than the tempo any student with ASD in the class chooses when using movement

for self-stimulation (e.g., rocking or spinning; Alvin, 1991). The increase in tempo helps the child become more aware of the environment outside his or her inner world.

- Emphasize repetition.
- Provide multiple opportunities for students to complete activities that incorporate only one movement; only then move to activities that require completion of a sequence of movements.
- To address problems with motor planning, teach movement sequences in small chunks, with sufficient time spent learning a segment or portion before performing the full sequence of movements.
- Suit movements to the imagery of songs.
- Choose instrumental pieces that lend themselves to concrete ideas for movements.
- Create multiple avenues for children to model aural and/or visual images through movement.
- Props such as balls or hula hoops provide a visual focus for movement activities, helping students to perform with appropriate energy or force (e.g., tempo, weight).
- Intersperse activities in which all students imitate the leader's movements (e.g., all participants raise and lower their arms to show the beat) with activities in which students create their own movement (e.g., children pretend they are dinosaurs).
- Hand-over-hand assistance may help children perform movements in beginning stages (e.g., when participants raise and lower arms to show the beat, a teacher, instructional assistant, or peer stands in front of the child with ASD and gently raises and lowers the child's arms).
- Supplement verbal directions with photographs or illustrations.
- Children on the autism spectrum may not know what they are supposed to focus on when asked to watch a live model, so supplement visual models with simple verbal directions as to where they should pay particular attention (Staples & Reid, 2010).

Nonlocomotor movement

Nonlocomotor refers to an individual's movements while sitting or standing in place. Children may engage in nonlocomotor movements on their own or with a partner. Nonlocomotor movements commonly taught in music classrooms and descriptions of these movements are listed in Table 5.4. The activities that follow provide children with opportunities to practice nonlocomotor movements.

TABLE 5.4

Non-Locomotor Movements

Movement	Description
bend/curl	Flex the body forward bringing upper and lower body parts together. A bend or curl from a sitting position on the floor is easier than from a standing position as it is easier to balance the body when sitting.
stretch	Bring arms over head and extend as high as possible. Feet can be flat on the floor or, in stretching, the individual may rise up on the tips of the toes.
swing	Make large front and back (back and forth) movements, usually with the arms.
bounce	Flex and straighten the legs, propelling the feet off the floor, then return to the first position.
shake	Tremble or shiver. This movement could engage the whole body or portions of the body (e.g., shake your left hand).
shoulder shrugs	Move shoulders up toward base of skull and then back to a natural standing position.
sway	Swing but with smaller motions.
straight	Make straight movements.
round	Similarly to a bend or curl, flex the head, neck, and upper back over the lower body creating a rounded shape.
levels: high, middle, low	Low movements occur at the level of the feet or legs; middle-level movements occur at the level of the waist and chest; high movements occur at the level of the head or above.
turn	Change the direction the body faces. In a quarter turn, the body moves from the facing direction to face either side (a quarter turn to the left or the right); In a full turn, the body moves 180 degrees to face the opposite direction.
narrow/wide	Legs and/or arms are held close to the body; Legs and/or arms are held away from the body.

(Adapted, in part, from Boswell, 2005)

These activities rely, in large part, on building skills in imitation. This section begins with body awareness and body exploration exercises that are ideal warm-up or cool-down exercises for many educational enterprises and are especially well-suited to music classes where imitation of simple movements helps to build the student's innate sense of beat and rhythm. The teacher models movements demonstrating a comfortable and relaxed tempo. When introducing simple movement activities teachers may wish to begin with movements using both sides of the body (bilateral coordination); for example, students put both hands on hips (see Figure 5.2, top frame). Later, movements may use only one side of the body (unilateral coordination); for example, holding one arm out in front of the body (see Figure 5.2, middle frame). Some of the motions, such as "shake your whole

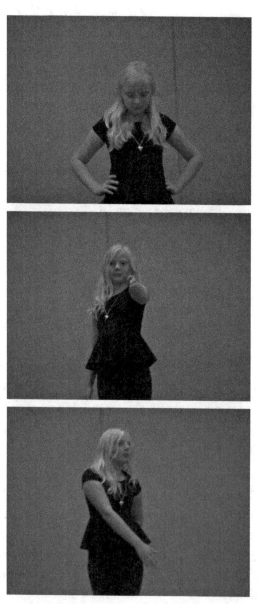

FIGURE 5.2 Bilateral (top), Unilateral (middle), and Cross-Lateral (bottom) Movements

body," suggest a standing posture. When motions can be completed equally well sitting or standing (e.g., "tap your head") children may be asked to sit as this position requires less attention to balance than standing. Motions that cross the midline, such as moving one arm across the front of the body may be introduced after children have demonstrated some confidence in unilateral motions (see Figure 5.2, bottom frame). Integrating sequences of movements comes after children have gained some control over their movements by performing single motions in isolation, have demonstrated the ability to follow the leader's directions, and have acquired a movement vocabulary.

Students on the autism spectrum often have difficulties judging the force or weight of their movements. Nonlocomotor activities provide students with opportunities to explore how they can control the energy or effort of their movements and how changes to the energy or effort affect the movements. Educators can encourage this experimentation by asking students to vary the force of their movements, for example, by moving their arms lightly or making heavy movements with their legs. They can vary the tempo by contrasting fast movements with slow movements. They can change the flow by contrasting smooth with jagged movements.

Children on the autism spectrum might not be able to copy the teacher's actions as soon as movement activities are presented. The same behaviors might be observed here as in other activities ranging from resisting to ignoring, to engaging, to actively participating (see Chapter 4, pages 112 to 113 for a more complete description of these behaviors in the context of the scarf game).

Instructional interventions
SPACE AWARENESS (ADAPTED FROM WOOD, 1996). Wood (1996) suggests a variety of ways in which children may explore their sense of personal space. Some of her advice is listed below, with ideas for involving children with ASD.

- Find your own space. Personal spaces may be marked visually by using carpet squares or tape on the floor (if this is allowed by school administration and/or custodians). When working with groups of students, teachers often establish a routine in which children quietly enter the room. Depending on the particular group, this routine might be highly structured so that each student goes to a particular place in the room. In a less structured environment, each student is free to find any space (e.g., carpet square) in the room, so long as there is one student in each place (unless the particular activities require students to work in pairs or groups).
- Sit or stand in the space. Whether the students sit or stand in the space depends on the background experience and/or age of the children, keeping

in mind that exploring the space in a standing position requires greater attention to balance.

- Feel all around the space with your arms. Students may stretch arms over their heads, hold their arms out to their sides, and in front of or behind their bodies. They observe where their space begins (at the core of the body) and ends (as far as the arms can reach). They observe where other people's spaces begin and end.
- Start by standing in place. Move away from this starting point, circle around it, and then return to the original place. This provides a sense of freedom to the movements by showing the students that they do not always need to face in the same direction. If particular students like to twirl in circles for self stimulation, teachers may omit this type of space exploration.
- Kick feet out of the space (one at a time), feeling how this changes the students' balance.

This is not an exhaustive list. Teachers and students are encouraged to work together to find additional ways for children to experiment with the area within their personal spaces.

BODY AWARENESS. The teacher names parts of the body and demonstrates a motion. For example, the teacher nods his or her head while playing a pattern on the drum, repeating a quarter note followed by a quarter rest (Figure 5.3). ▶

Movements reflect this pattern with the teacher moving a body part while playing the quarter note and coming back to the starting position on the rest. To create consistency between this activity and the activities that follow, teachers view this pattern as an 8-beat phrase as this models the phrase length common to many children's songs. The teacher repeats this pattern until the students have sufficient opportunity to mirror the teacher's actions. It is not necessarily expected that students' motions will reflect the pattern played on the drum as soon as students are first introduced to this activity. This skill is refined through practice. As students gain experience, their movements more closely follow the sounds produced on the drum. The duration (number of beats) for each segment of the activity will depend on the students' readiness to participate.

Notation for 8-Beat Phrase for Body Awareness Game

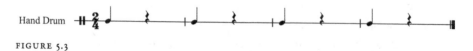

FIGURE 5.3

As illustrated in Figure 5.4, students may perform a variety of movements:

a. Nod Head
b. Open Mouth
c. Shoulder Shrug
d. Leg Lift
e. Stretch

- Head Nods: Relate the motions to commonly used meaningful gestures such as gently nodding the head up and down to indicate "yes" or moving the head gently from side to side to indicate "no" (Figure 5.4, frame a). To correspond to the sounds of the drum, the teacher moves his or her head to the right on the quarter note and back to the starting position on the rest; then moves the head to the left on the next quarter note and back to the starting position for the rest.
- Mouths: Open and close mouths (Figure 5.4, frame b).
- Shoulder Shrugs: Lift shoulders towards ears and return to the starting position; roll shoulders forward and return to the starting position (Figure 5.1, frame c); roll shoulders back and return to the starting position (Heutig, Pyfer, & Auxter, 2001).
- Leg Lifts: Lift one leg off the floor by bending the leg at the hip and allowing the knee to bend, return to the starting position; lift the other leg off the floor by bending the leg at the hip and allowing the knee to bend, return to starting position (Figure 5.4, frame d).
- Stretches: Raise one arm over the head and bend the waist downward on the opposite side, return to starting position; raise the other arm over the head and bend the waist downward on the opposite side, return to starting position (Figure 5.4, frame e);

FULL BODY MOVEMENTS IN PLACE. Full body movements in place may be approached as a move and freeze game. The children move when the teacher plays an instrument (such as a hand drum). The teacher might explain to the students that this is the *magic drum* or the *talking drum* and that they must listen carefully and follow the drum's directions. Students move their bodies when they hear quarter notes; the dotted eighth–sixteenth note pattern on beat 7 is their cue to freeze (Figure 5.5). This aural cue is well suited to children on the autism spectrum as they have opportunities to follow directions that do not rely on verbal communication.

While Figure 5.5 illustrates an 8-beat phrase, in practice the length of the pattern is changed to *surprise* the students as they listen and respond to what they hear. ▶

Motivation is added to the game by asking children to freeze in various positions. For example:

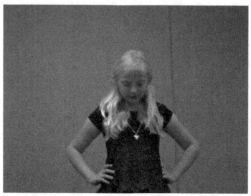

(a) not head

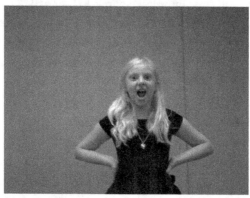

(b) open mouth

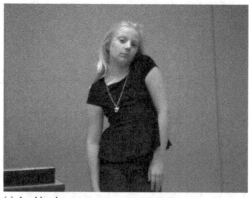

(c) shoulder shrug

FIGURE 5.4 Continued

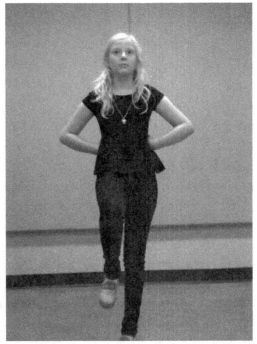

(d) leg lift

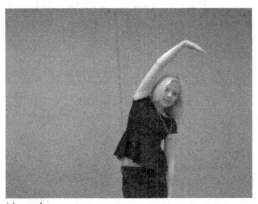

(e) stretch

FIGURE 5.4 Movements to Promote Body Awareness

- Shake your whole body; freeze like a giraffe.
- Shake your whole body; freeze like a mouse.

Students do not need to move their bodies to reflect the beat of the drum. Rather, the purpose of this game is for the students to gain comfort in moving their bodies

Notation for Nonlocomotor Freeze Game

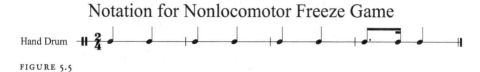

FIGURE 5.5

and learn to respond to the directions of the drum. They will have plenty of opportunities to reflect specific beat and rhythm through movement in more advanced activities.

MOVEMENT AND RECORDED MUSIC. Nonlocomotor movements may be accompanied by recorded music. Guidelines for choosing recorded music are consistent with specifications outlined in Chapter 4: Listening to Music.

MOVE AND FREEZE. This intervention is similar to the activity in which children move their bodies while the teacher plays a drum and students freeze their movements on the given signal. In this intervention, though, the teacher plays recorded music. While sitting or standing in place, students move their bodies in ways that reflect the character of the music; they stop moving (freeze) when the teacher stops the music and continue to move when the teacher starts the music again. As with previous games in music, students on the autism spectrum have opportunities to demonstrate their ability to listen and follow directions without relying on verbal instructions.

This activity provides avenues for students to continue practicing their control of the effort and energy in their movements as, with ongoing experience, their motions increasingly reflect the character of the music. Fast music may inspire quick, jagged, and tense movements; slow music may inspire large, smooth, and relaxed motions. Quiet music may inspire small and gentle movement; loud music may encourage large movements. Music with jagged melodies may bring forth jagged body movements while music with long flowing, step-wise motion may transfer to long, smooth, flowing movements from the students. Selections of recorded music suited to this activity are provided in Tables 5.5 and 5.6 to assist teachers in implementing this activity in their classrooms. Readers are encouraged to expand this list with their own selections, noting which music best motivates their students to take part in the educational interventions outlined here.

ROLL THE BALL. For this activity, students on the autism spectrum work with partners, generally an educational assistant or a peer. The participants sit on the floor facing each other with their legs open in front of them in the shape of the letter V. Children are sufficiently close to each other so they can roll the ball back and

TABLE 5.5

Freeze Game: Western Art Music

Composer	Artist(s)	Title	Duration	Album	Label
Albinoni	London Virtuosi (John Georgiadis)	Concerto in F major, op. 9, no. 5 (movement 2 – adagio non troppo)	2:11	Albinoni Oboe Concerti	Naxos
Ravel	Trio Verlaine	Prelude pour piano	1'16	Trio Verlaine	Skylark
				Fin de siècle: The music of Debussy and Ravel	
Ravel	Trio Verlaine	Le Tombeau de Couperin (fugue)	4'00	Trio Verlaine	Skylark
				Fin de siècle: The music of Debussy and Ravel	
Vivaldi	Orchestra de camera "I Filarmonici" (Albertao Martini)	Concerto No. 4 in E minor RV550	2'20	Vivaldi Masterworks	Brilliant Classics

TABLE 5.6

Freeze Game: Jazz

Artist	Title	Duration	Album	Label	Catalog number
Botti, C.	Night Sessions	3:43	Streets Ahead	Columbia	CK 85753
Jobim, A. C.	Corcovado	2:16	The Essential Antonio Carlos Jobim	Verve	836 253-2
Sinclaire, D.	This is My Lucky Day	2:47	Denzal Sinclaire	Verve	4400385782
Sinclaire, D.	The Art of Living	3:54	Denzal Sinclaire	Verve	4400385782
Sinclaire, D.	A Peaceful Soul	4:11	Denzal Sinclaire	Verve	4400385782
Sinclaire, D.	Still Got It	1:16	Denzal Sinclaire	Verve	4400385782
Wright, L.	Wake Up, Little Sparrow	3:01	Dreaming Wide Awake	Verve Forecast	8000406902

forth in the space outlined by their legs but far enough away from each other so their feet do not touch. Children listen to music while they roll the ball back and forth. For suggested recordings see Tables 5.7 and 5.8.

When I first introduced this activity, I envisioned students rolling balls back and forth to reflect the beat of the music. While these students were able to recognize and reflect the beat in their movements, this competency did not transfer to the ball rolling activity. The music is foundational, however, as it cues the beginning and the ending of the activity.

This ball rolling game contributes to programming for students on the autism spectrum because it encourages collaborative behaviors and joint attention. It is a viable way for students to practice the reach-to-grasp response (Hughes, 1996; Lawson, 2003; Mari et al., 2003), employing skills such as visual perception (in judging the location of the ball), reaching toward the ball (with the arm), grasping the ball (with the hands), and exerting sufficient energy (to return the ball to the partner).

This game may be adapted to address particular issues of specific children. For example, if a child is reluctant to sit on the floor, the partners may gently toss or bounce the ball back and forth while sitting across from each other in chairs. As well

TABLE 5.7

Ball Passing: Western Art Music

Composer	Artist(s)	Title	Duration	Album	Label	Catalog number
Chopin, F.	Janusz Olejniczak	Mazurka in F minor op. 68, no. 4	3:04	Chopin: Janusz Olejniczak Polonezy Mazurki Nokturny	Fryderyk Chopin Institute	none
Mozart, W. A.	Academy of St Martin in the Fields (Sir Neville Marriner)	Symphony #28 in C, KV200/189k (Movement 3: Menueto [Allegretto])	3:52	Complete Mozart Edition (Symphonies 21–33) (volume 2, cd 2)	Philips	422 613-2
Mozart, W. A.	Academy of St. Martin in the Fields	Symphony #24 in B flat, KV182/173d (Movement 3: Allegro)	3:02	Complete Mozart Edition (Symphonies 21–33) (volume 2, cd 1)	Phillips	422 612-2
Poulenc, F.	Alexandre Tharaud, piano; Thibault Viex, violin; Ronald Van Spaendonck, clarinet; Stephane Logerot, double bass	L'invitation au Chateau, movement de valse	1:32	Complete Chamber Music, volume 5	Naxos	8.553611F
Ravel, M.	Trio Verlaine	Sonatine	2:32	Fin de Siècle: The music of Debussy and Ravel	Skylark	none

TABLE 5.8

Ball Passing: Jazz

Artist	Title	Duration	Album	Label	Catalog number
Botti, C.	Lisa	5:08	Night Sessions	Columbia	CK 85753
George Shearing Quintet	Let It Snow	6:20	Christmas with the George Shearing Quintet	Telarc	83438

if the children are standing across from each other, the distance and the number of times the ball bounces can be adjusted to fit the age, experience, and proficiency of the students.

IMITATING MOVEMENTS. Recorded music provides a foundation for imitation through movement. In music classes, students often engage in an activity called "the mirrors game". In this game, students become mirrors, imitating the leader's (often the teacher) actions. The teacher devises movements that fit the character of the music (e.g., force, tempo, flow [see Table 5.2]). Taking into account the difficulties experienced by children with ASD when expected to imitate another's actions, students may begin this activity using easier bilateral movements before advancing to more difficult unilateral and cross lateral motions. For example, students mirror motions in which they raise both arms or bend both knees (bilateral) before mirroring motions in which they raise one arm (unilateral) or motions in which the left arm reaches across the vertical mid-line of the body (cross lateral). As well, students begin imitating motions while seated, graduating to motions from a standing position when they are able to maintain a stable posture.

In recognition that individuals with ASD experience difficulties with motor planning, students might be introduced to this game by imitating a single motion throughout the entire piece. They might then be introduced to a simple movement sequence: for example, the students might raise and lower both arms above their heads and then raise their arms in front of their bodies. This sequence continues for the duration of the piece. If children have difficulties performing a sequence of movements, teachers might use gentle physical guidance, such as hand-over-hand instruction, along with verbal explanations of each sequence of the task (Bhat et al., 2011).

When more complicated unilateral or cross lateral movements are added, teachers emphasize that the children mirror the leader's motions. The teacher, who generally faces the students, decides on the sequence the students perform and adjusts the

(a) 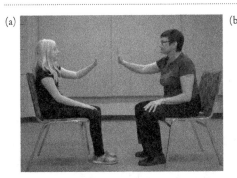 (b)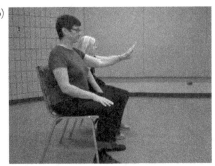

FIGURE 5.6 Imitating Partner: Facing (left) and Beside (right)

given visual to account for reversal. For example, if the sequence begins with the children lifting their left arms, the teacher moves his or her right (see Figure 5.6: left frame). Alternately, the leader (or designate) could sit or stand beside the student (Todd, 2012). From this position, the student does not need to mirror actions, but moves the same part of the body as the leader. For example, both the teacher and the student raise their left arms (see Figure 5.6: right frame). The down side of this approach is that social communication may be inhibited when the individuals are not able to face (and look at) each other.

In a variation on this game, motions are completed while participants hold props such as streamers or scarves. Students may be motivated to take part in this activity because they can choose a scarf in their favorite color. As well, props provide a visual cue to the movement and therefore may help the students with their visual perception. Props are used judiciously due to possible drawbacks. First, there is a potential for the child's attention to the prop to supersede attention to the presenter, thereby limiting joint attention. Second, the props may provide visual stimulation that draws students away from the game. For example, a student may become so engaged in the bright flashes of light produced by metallic streamers that the prop intended as a motivational tool for engagement becomes a tool for self-stimulation.

Locomotor movement

Many children with ASD find it challenging to perform locomotor tasks. They tend to walk at a slower pace than their typically developing peers, with smaller strides and less movement in their arms (Bhat, et al., 2011). They tend to have difficulties coordinating their head, shoulders, and pelvis during locomotion (Vernazza-Martin et al., 2005). As well, they have difficulties coordinating arm movements when running (Morin & Reid, 1985). Children on the autism spectrum benefit from structured activities that guide their practice toward greater skills in locomotion.

The acquisition of skills in movement is not viewed as a hierarchy in which children achieve excellence in performing motions in place (nonlocomotor) before engaging in structured activities to gain competence in moving through space (locomotor). Students' acquisition of movement skills begins with non-locomotor movements to prepare readiness for the more challenging locomotor tasks. When students begin to develop accuracy with nonlocomotor motions and demonstrate understanding of the basic movement vocabulary by respond-ing correctly to verbal directions, they are ready to begin engagements with loco-motor movements (see Table 5.9). Nonlocomotor and locomotor movements are then explored at the same time, with the teacher and/or students choos-ing the type of motions that best suit the given activities. Thus, students are practicing and refining a variety of nonlocomotor and locomotor movements concurrently.

Instructional interventions

Activities in which children walk through space offer many benefits. Students are encouraged to walk the beat of the music (provided by the teacher and/or in record-ings). This promotes the coordination of movements at a steady tempo. For students

TABLE 5.9

Locomotor Movements	
Movement	Description
gallop	The fast gait of a horse when all four feet are off the ground; in music class, to gallop is to imitate such a gait by leaping with uneven strides.
glide/slide	To move feet smoothly across the floor.
hop	A hop can be performed on two legs or one. For a two-legged hop, the body springs upward as both feet leave the floor simultaneously in a leaping motion; in a one-legged hop, a one-legged hop is performed with one leg held off the ground, the body springs upward as the supporting foot leaves the floor in a leaping motion
run	Propel the body forward with steady equidistant strides at a quicker pace than a walk; a sprint is faster than a run; a jog is slow than a sprint but faster than a run.
skip	A gait alternating a step and a hop on one foot with a step and a hop on the other foot.
walk	Propel the body forward with steady equidistant strides.

on the autism spectrum, this steady tempo can influence gait. The teacher's beat provides an aural cue to the initiation and completion of each step. This helps the students produce strides of equal length. By walking to various tempi, students control the length of their strides. This provides them with practice in controlling and coordinating their body as they move through space.

THE MAGIC DRUM/THE TALKING DRUM. Students are motivated to create full body movements through space with the *magic drum* (also called the *talking drum*). In this activity, students listen to the drum and move through the open classroom space when the drum tells them to move and freeze when the drum tells them to freeze (stop moving and hold your position). This activity is illustrated in Figure 5.7.

This section begins with a description of a walking pattern, followed by variations that include running, sliding, hopping, and skipping.[1] For each motion, notation is provided for 8- and 16-beat phrases to assist teachers in creating the rhythmic patterns that the students model through their actions. Aural examples are included on the companion website.

1. Walk

Using the *magic drum* the teacher plays 8 beats on the drum. The first 6 beats are quarter notes, beat 7 is a dotted-eighth–sixteenth-note pattern that signals students to freeze on the quarter note that follows on beat 8 (see Figure 5.5). This pattern may be extended to 16 beats (see Figure 5.8). This pattern is familiar to the students from

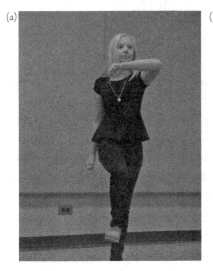
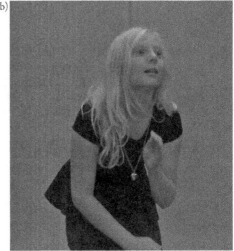

FIGURE 5.7 March (left) and Freeze (right)

Notation for Locomotor Freeze Game (16 beats): Walking

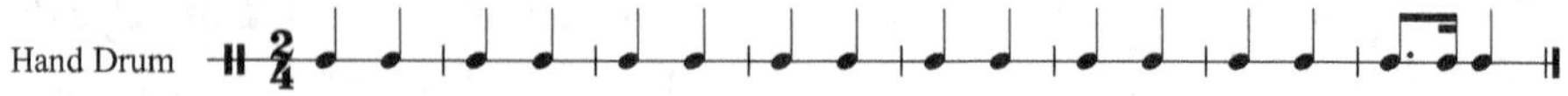

FIGURE 5.8

the nonlocomotor freeze game using the *magic drum* that was described earlier in this chapter. I use a hand drum for this activity. Non-pitched percussion instruments such as claves, rhythm sticks, and wood blocks work as well. ▶ ▶

The teacher cues the beginning of the activity with a four-beat spoken introduction such as "One, Two, Here We Go." This phrase provides children with the tempo for the activity. Children walk to the beat, freezing on the signal provided by the drum (dotted-eighth–sixteenth-note pattern).

The formation of the students around the classroom's open space varies depending on the number of children in the class and the space available. Ideally, there is sufficient open space for them to move freely through the space while negotiating objects and other people in the room. Teachers should provide instructions as to any areas of the room that are not available for student exploration (e.g., the area behind the teacher's desk). If feasible, the free space may be marked on the floor with tape, choosing a color that is visible with ease. In beginning activities, Wood (1995) suggests that all children move counterclockwise. This reduces the possibility that students will walk into each other. As well, the activity seems less daunting as children are not concerned that people will approach them from all directions. This promotes collaboration and a sense that all children are a part of the group. It also provides them with opportunities to become familiar with the physical shape and size of the room. All students are encouraged to participate and, in the beginning stages of musical development, participation is more important than the accuracy of the movements (Wood, 1995).

As children gain facility with this activity, they choose the directions in which they walk through free space. Many of the variations below lend themselves to this approach. Children might also practice walking in lines or circles. These approaches are more difficult because they require an increased awareness of and ability to negotiate the space in relation to others.

After children demonstrate some facility and comfort walking as described above, the teacher may choose to modify the basic activity. Many children need a great deal of practice to master locomotion. The variations provide students with opportunities to refine the basic walk and to control their bodies in different ways depending on how they are instructed to walk. Children do not need to coordinate their movements with the drum perfectly before incorporating the variations. The variations provide additional practice in walking, adding elements that challenge students to control their movements. As well, many of these activities provide children with opportunities to communicate their ideas in creative ways.

> Variation 1: Students perform a basic walk and freeze their bodies in shapes suggested by the leader: for example, straight, bent or curled, reaching high, touching toes, crouching low, arms extended from body, or arms held close to body. In this activity students demonstrate understanding of the movement vocabulary acquired during the nonlocomotor activities and apply this understanding in combination with walking and reacting to the aural cue to freeze.
>
> Variation 2: Students vary the energy of their walking steps. For example, the body is bent over and the weight of the steps is heavy as they pretend they are carrying a stack of books or the steps are light and the body is buoyant if they pretend they are carrying a feather. Viewing the objects will help students on the autism spectrum to imagine the relative weight of the motions.
>
> Variation 3: Students vary the direction in which they travel, following the teacher's directions and moving forward, backward, sideways, in a straight line, or in a zigzag. Students negotiate these movements with a partner, holding hands or, if this creates sensory challenges for students with ASD, standing side-by-side.
>
> Variation 4: Students move their bodies into shapes suggested by the teacher as they walk, and freeze. For example, they form a large shape with legs and arms wide from the body or form a narrow shape with legs and arms held close to the body (Boswell, 2005).
>
> Variation 5: The teacher plays ascending and descending scale patterns on the piano (see Figure 5.9). When the tones gradually sound higher the students walk forward, when the notes gradually sound lower the students walk backward (Montgomery, 2002). Using this technique, students demonstrate awareness of pitch and changes in pitch without being limited to, or requiring, a verbal response. ⊙

Notation for Walking Forward and Backward

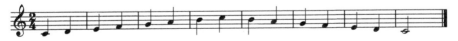

FIGURE 5.9

2. Run

When leading movement activities with the *magic drum* the beats are quarter notes (walking) and subdivisions of the beats into two equal parts are eighth notes (running). The teacher models running on the balls of the feet rather than the heel-to-toe pattern of steps and encourages the students to model his or her movements (Wood, 1995). As well, the teacher explains that there are two running steps in the same time period as one walking step. Because of this, running steps are approximately half the length of a walking step.

Children perform the same activities described for walking, but this time the teacher plays eighth notes, ending with the same cue to stop or freeze (see Figures 5.10 and 5.11). ▶ ▶

The teacher can also vary the sounds, sometimes playing the eight-beat phrase using quarter notes and sometimes playing the eight-beat phrase using eighth notes. Children walk when they hear quarter notes (one sound on one beat) and run when they hear eighth notes (two equal sounds on one beat).

3. Slide

Using the *magic drum* sliding movements reflect half notes (one sound on two beats). The teacher models this by striking the drum and sliding the hand across the drum for two-beats. This provides the students with an aural guide to the length of the slide. The teacher models a sliding motion, putting weight on the right leg and sliding the left foot across the floor for two beats, then alternating the movement with weight on the left leg and sliding the right foot. Students mirror this action,

Notation for Locomotor Freeze Game (8 beats): Running

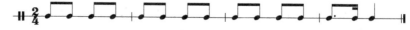

FIGURE 5.10

Notation for Locomotor Freeze Game (16 beats): Running

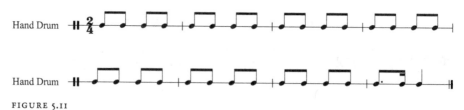

FIGURE 5.11

beginning the sliding motions with the foot they choose. The teacher compares steps and slides, explaining that two staps require the same amount of time as one slide.

Students perform the same activities described for walking and running, but this time the teacher plays sliding sounds for the first two measures of a four-measure pattern, or six measures of an eight-measure pattern, ending the phrase with a dotted-quarter–eighth-note pattern as the signal to stop (see Figures 5.12 and 5.13). ⏵ ⏵

The teacher can also vary the sounds, sometimes playing quarter notes (walking), sometimes playing eighth notes (running), and sometimes playing half notes (sliding). Students change their motions to reflect what they hear.

4. Hop

Using the *magic drum,* hopping movements reflect a quarter note followed by a quarter rest (see Figures 5.14 and 5.15). ⏵ ⏵

The teacher models the difference between a half note and a quarter note followed by a quarter rest by striking the drum on beat one and moving the hand away from the drum for beat two. The teacher models a two-legged hop, placing feet close together, flexing the knees, and springing the body upward while both feet leave the floor simultaneously. Depending on the expertise of the students, they could hop upward and

Notation for Locomotor Freeze Game (8 beats) Sliding

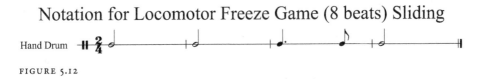

FIGURE 5.12

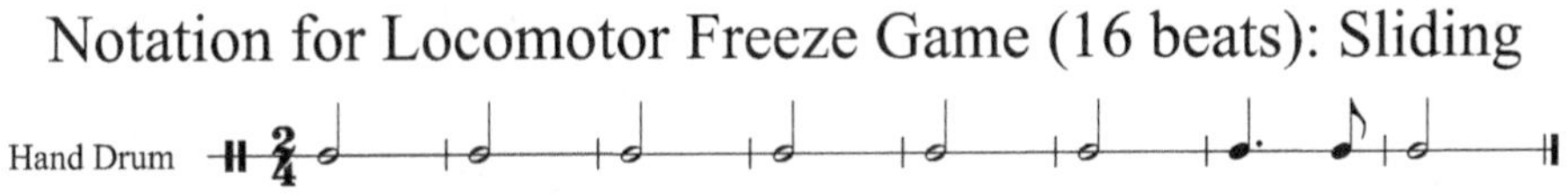

Notation for Locomotor Freeze Game (16 beats): Sliding

FIGURE 5.13

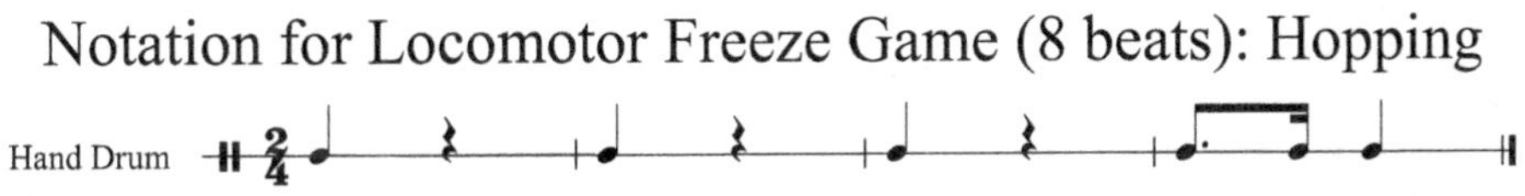

Notation for Locomotor Freeze Game (8 beats): Hopping

FIGURE 5.14

Notation for Locomotor Freeze Game (16 beats): Hopping

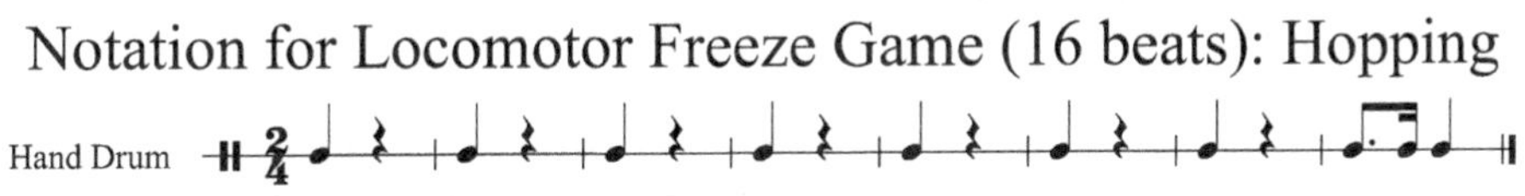

FIGURE 5.15

land on the same spot or they could use their arms to build forward momentum to propel the body forward. A line taped across the floor can act as a visual marker with the students hopping on the line or back and forth across the line (Heutig et al., 2001).

The teacher can vary the sounds, sometimes playing quarter notes (walking), sometimes playing eighth notes (running), sometimes playing half notes (sliding), and sometimes playing quarter notes followed by a rest (hopping). Students change their motions to reflect what they hear.

5. Skip

Skipping motions differ from the previous movements because the meter is compound (6/8) instead of simple (2/4); see Figures 5.16 and 5.17). These figures are denoted as 8 and 16 beat measures when each beat equals a dotted quarter note. The teacher taps the quarter notes and eighth notes on the drum and models the step (quarter note) and hop (eighth note) motion required for skipping (e.g., alternating step and hop on the right foot and step and hop on the left foot). ▶ ▶

The teacher can vary the sounds, sometimes playing quarter notes (walking), sometimes playing eighth notes (running), sometimes playing half notes (sliding), sometimes playing quarter notes followed by quarter rests (hopping), and sometimes playing quarter notes followed by eighth notes (skipping). Students change their motions to reflect what they hear.

FREE DANCING. In this activity, students interact with the learning community in a semi-structured activity where all participants (teacher, instructional assistants, and students) dance as suggested by the character of the music. In my classes, this activity is generally placed at the end of a session with up-tempo selections that

Notation for Locomotor Freeze Game (8 beats): Skipping

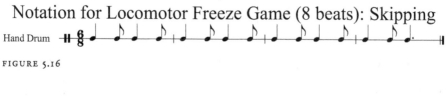

FIGURE 5.16

Notation for Locomotor Freeze Game (16 beats): Skipping

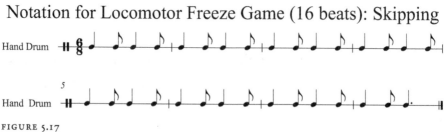

FIGURE 5.17

inspire children to leave their chairs and increase their levels of energy as the class comes to a close. This is an ideal forum to work on joint attention, with educational assistants crouching to the eye levels of the students and engaging them through movement, sometimes imitating how the children move and sometimes surprising them with unexpected motions (see also in Chapter 6: Instrumental Conversations Using Rhythm Sticks). When appropriate to the chosen music, participants have the option of playing non-pitched percussion instruments such as cluster bells or maracas. Recordings suitable for this activity are listed in Table 5.10.

Movement and Meter

Children gain an understanding of meter by moving in ways that reflect the patterns of accented and unaccented beats in music. For example, students might move from side to side to demonstrate metrical groups of 3 by moving in one direction for one strong beat and two weak beats and then move in the other direction for one strong beat and two weak beats. Students may also step in place to demonstrate metrical groups in 2. While some students seem to respond to meter naturally, many individuals require guidance and modeling to do so.

In the activity described here hula hoops are used as props. Students are grouped in partners. The structure of these pairs depends on the specifics of the classroom. The key is that one of the partners needs to have a strong sense of beat and meter. This person becomes the group leader, guiding the partner to move in ways that correspond to the meter of the music. If children with ASD are paired with a particular instructional assistant throughout the school day, this person might be the student's partner. If working in an inclusive environment, a student with ASD may partner with an instructional assistant or a peer.

Partners sit across from each other, with each partner grasping the opposite side of the hula hoop. Each set of partners has a group leader and partner designated as the follower. As the music begins, the group leader sways the hula hoop to the left and to the right, changing directions to reflect the meter of the music. For example, if the pattern of accented and unaccented beats is grouped in 3's, the group leader sways to the left for three beats and to the right for the next three beats. These movements, alternating from the left to the right, are maintained for the duration of the piece (provided that the meter of the music does not change). Since both students are holding the hula hoop, the movements of the follower should shift in the direction of the leader. The extent to which this occurs depends, in part, on the follower's willingness to go along with the leader. Hula hoops are pliable. If the student displays some resistance to the movements, the leader is able to pull the hula hoop to either side to reflect the meter of the piece. As the interaction continues the follower may

TABLE 5.10

Free Dancing

Artist/composer	Title	Duration	Album	Label	Catalog number
Benson, G.	Love Remembers	5:43	Love Remembers	Warner Brothers	9 26685-2
Cole, N.	Soon	3:12	Ask a Woman Who Knows	Verve	3145897742
Evans, B.	Peri's Scope	3:15	Portrait in Jazz	Riverside	OJCCD-088-2
Jobim, A. C.	Samba de uma nota so	2:15	The essential Antonio Carolos Jobim	Verve	836 253-2
Jobim, A. C.	So Danco Samba	2:13	The essential Antonio Carolos Jobim	Verve	836 253-2
Mancini, H.	Baby Elephant Walk	2:42	The Best of Henri Mancini	BMG Belgium	PA761/7
McDonald, M.	Mercy, Mercy Me	3:32	Motown 2	Motown	B000347202
Richie, L.	All Night Long	6:25	Can't Slow Down	Motown	37463 6059-2
Sinclaire, D.	This is My Lucky Day	2:47	Denzal Sinclaire	Verve	4400385782
Sinclaire, D.	Tofu and Greens	2:25	Denzal Sinclaire	Verve	4400385782

begin to move his or her arms or body in response to the motions of the leader. This activity may be put aside if resistance becomes too great, with the follower controlling the movements in ways that do not reflect the tempo or the meter of the music or throwing the hula hoop across the room.

After students become accustomed to the activity and are able to follow the leaders' motions from side-to-side, the leader may experiment with other motions that reflect the meter. Given that students on the autism spectrum have difficulty performing movement sequences, leaders might maintain a single motion throughout a listening session (perhaps moving the hula hoop up and down or side-to-side throughout the activity). More advanced routines may be devised that involve a sequence of movements.

Suggested musical selections to accompany this activity are provided in Table 5.11. In this Table, meter is denoted as groups of two beats or three beats in six selections from overtures composed by J. S. Bach. When used with this activity, three of the selections provide an impetus for moving the hula hoop back and forth in beat groupings of two, an accented beat followed by an unaccented beat. The other three selections provide an incentive for moving the hula hoop to reflect groups of three beats, an accented beat followed by two unaccented beats. Tempos are relative approximations and may vary in relation to the recorded version of these works chosen by the teacher. In practice, students engage in this activity while listening to a variety of tempi. The teacher takes note of the tempi of repetitive behaviors demonstrated by students with ASD, and chooses music that is faster than their natural predilections to urge them to engage with the tempo of their partners' movements.

Chapter Summary

In general, children on the autism spectrum display deficits in motor performance, with greater challenges in functioning observed in children at the severe end of the spectrum (Hardy & LaGasse, 2013). Difficulties emerge in several aspects of motor learning including gait and coordination, motor planning, the use of tools or objects, and the imitation of another's actions (LaGasse & Hardy, 2013).

Researchers conclude that individuals with ASD have fewer opportunities than their typically developing peers to refine motor function (e.g., Bhat et al., 2011). The educational interventions described here are approached through a sense of play in which students with ASD gain facility by engaging with others in interactive games derived around music. By engaging in these games, students gain an innate understanding of beat, rhythm, and meter in music. These aural cues help children to coordinate their movements with the beat, with accents that group beats into equal groupings, and with rhythm patterns that elongate or subdivide the beat.

TABLE 5.11

Movement and Meter: Bach Overtures

Title	Duration	Groupings of beats	Tempo
Overture No. 1 BWV 1066 in C major: 4. Forlane	1:13	3	*allegro* (fast)
Overture No. 1 BWV 1066 in C major: 6. Bouree I/II	2:21	2	*allegro* (fast)/*moderato* (moderate)/*allegro* (fast)
Overture No. 1 BWV 1066 in C major: 7. Passepied I/II	2:25	3	*andante* (moderately slow)
Overture No. 2 BWV 1067 in B minor: 2. Rondeau	1:58	2	*moderato* (moderate)
Overture No. 2 BWV 1067 in B minor: 4. Bouree I/II	1:57	2	*allegro* (fast)
Overture No. 2 BWV 1067 in B minor: 6. Menuet	1:31	3	*andante* (moderately slow)

Note: All pieces on this table are available on the recording *Johann Sebastian Bach: 6 Brandenburg Concertos/4 Orchestral Suites (Overtures)* by The English Consort, ARCHIV D284161."

Educational interventions in music provide avenues for students with ASD to improve gross and fine motors skills, balance, posture, imitation, and joint attention while engaging in activities that integrate music and movement. Music education provides opportunities for students to acquire skills related to body awareness (how the body moves), and spatial awareness (how the body moves in place or through space). Students also explore effort or energy (force, speed, and weight), and relationships (moving alone, with partners, or in groups) while playing the musical games described in this chapter (Buschner, 1994). The increased ease of mobility that students with ASD gain through practice in this educational environment has the potential to affect how they interact in other environments, both at school (e.g., on the playground) or in their lives outside of school (e.g., playing with siblings). From this perspective, music and music education have the potential to positively impact the quality of life for students with ASD.

Discussion Questions

1. What motor challenges are typically encountered by children with ASD?
2. How do students with ASD benefit from educational experiences that combine motor responses with music.

3. What are the steps in motor planning required of students to complete the motor tasks they typically encounter in their day-to-day lives (e.g., getting dressed, eating, and traveling to school).

4. What are the steps in motor planning required for students to complete motor tasks typically encountered in school.

Note

1. This activity emerges from educational strategies developed by Emile Jaques-Dalcroze, namely, the quick reaction, in which students devise movements in response to what they hear (Abramson 1997; Choksy et al. 2001). Wood (1996) is recommended for teachers searching for additional movement games.

6

PLAYING MUSICAL INSTRUMENTS

BY PLAYING MUSICAL instruments, students enhance their competencies in music and build their understanding of the fundamental concepts of music, especially those associated with beat and rhythm. Non-pitched percussion instruments (e.g., hand drums, rhythm sticks, and triangles) provide students with hands-on experiences in making music without requiring extensive musical skills (Nordoff & Robbins, 2007). Students with autism spectrum disorder receive many benefits from participating in music through playing musical instruments. The pleasure students with ASD gain from playing musical instruments motivates them to remain focused on current classroom activities. Successful experiences increase the students' motivation to learn through music and to interact with others in music-making activities. Successful experiences in music classes help students with ASD acquire a sense of accomplishment. This results in increased self-confidence and self-esteem through active participation (Nordoff & Robbins, 2007).

Playing instruments provides students with opportunities to learn how to recognize and respond appropriately to a variety of instrument timbres. This allows opportunities for students to adjust to those sounds that may cause overstimulation (e.g., the loud sounds of cow bells). As well, students have opportunities to choose the activities they will engage in by naming the instruments verbally or by miming the movements required for performance. This provides opportunities for students who are nonverbal, or who have limited verbal abilities, to actively choose what instruments they play. Playing instruments provides student with ASD who have limited verbal skills opportunities to engage in group music-making opportunities that do not rely on verbal abilities to engage in activities with their peers.

This chapter offers an overview of factors to consider when choosing instruments for particular tasks and for particular students are discussed:

1. Timbre or tone quality, based on materials of construction
2. How instruments are played
3. Ease of performance

This discussion is followed by guidelines for introducing percussion instruments to students and descriptions of educational interventions that facilitate the use of percussion instruments with students, highlighting how these strategies may be suited to students with autism spectrum disorder (ASD).

Categorizing Instruments

Three factors are discussed for choosing percussion instruments for educational interventions and for particular students to play: What materials instruments are made from, how instruments are played, and how easy instruments are to play.

MATERIALS OF CONSTRUCTION

Classroom percussion instruments are often categorized, by the materials used in their construction, as gourds, metals, skins, and woods (see Table 6.1). A fifth category is included here to denote instruments defined not so much by their materials as by their use to create sound effects.

This overview of percussion instruments includes all of the instruments used in the teaching interventions described in this book. For descriptions of the full range of music instruments used in elementary schools (both melodic and percussive) readers are directed to textbooks in music education (e.g., Berarducci, nd; Boyer & Rozmajlz, 2012; Campbell & Scott-Kassner, 2006; Montgomery, 2002). Readers interested in instruments adapted for students with special educational needs are directed to Darrow (2008).

Gourds (maracas and shakers)

Maracas originated in Latin America. Traditionally, they consisted of hollow balls made from dried gourds, commonly filled with seeds or dried beans, and attached

TABLE 6.1

Timbre or Tone Quality Based on Materials of Construction

gourds	metals	skins	woods
maracas	cymbals	drum	wood block
chikitas	finger cymbals		tick tock block
egg shakers	jingle bells		sand blocks
	cluster bells		rhythm sticks
	cowbell		claves
	agogo bells		guiro
	tambourine		
	triangle		
	cabasa		

to wooden handles. This explains their classification as gourds (see Figure 6.1). In general, instruments manufactured for use in elementary schools are constructed of wood or plastic. Most often a player grasps the handles, holds the instruments in front of the body, and shakes his or her arms and/or hands to create sounds. The sounds are varied by striking the instrument on the hands or legs.

Many variations of this instrument are available, including but not limited to chikitas, egg shakers, and twin chikitas (see Figure 6.1). Technically not gourds, they are described here because of their close association with maracas. Egg shakers are egg-shaped ovals. Players hold these in their palms and create sounds by shaking their hands. Chikitas are egg shakers attached to handles. They are played in the same manner as maracas. Twin chikitas are lengths of plastic with egg-type shakers at each end. To play, the student grasps the instrument in the middle, holds the instrument either vertically or horizontally and shakes his or her arm.

I find that students with ASD respond positively to shakers. The colors used in the manufacture of chikitas and egg shakers (blue, green, red, pink, and yellow) seem to motivate students to engage in classroom activities using these instruments. When given freedom over the choice of shakers, my students with ASD tend to prefer chikitas and twin chikitas to egg shakers.

Metals

Cymbals

Some students with ASD may dislike the sounds created by cymbals, so that this instrument choice may be more appropriate after students have had time and experience to adjust to the various sounds created by classroom percussion instruments. Cymbals are shallow round concave plates of thin metal (e.g., brass). In general, the

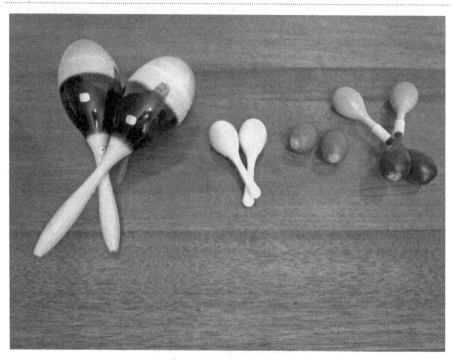

FIGURE 6.1 Maracas, Chikitas, Egg Shakers, and Twin Chikitas

cymbals created for young players are purchased in pairs (see Figure 6.2). Each cymbal has a hole drilled in its center that is fitted with a wooden handle or a leather strap. Typically, the player holds the cymbals vertically. The upper edge of one cymbal (designated here as the first cymbal) makes contact with the lower part of its partner (designated here as the second cymbal). The player then scrapes the first cymbal along the second cymbal using an upward motion with the hand that holds the first cymbal. Sets of cymbals vary in diameter allowing teachers to choose size and weight that best suit individual players.

Finger cymbals

Finger cymbals are miniature versions of full sized cymbals (see Figure 6.2). They have a small elastic loop attached in their center. Players place their index fingers inside the loops and press their thumbs against the outsides of the loops to form a secure hold on the instruments. Players hold the cymbals in front of themselves, one slightly above the other and overlapping slightly. The upper cymbal is moved downward to make contact with its partner. Challenges in placing fingers around the elastic loop create frustration for some students with ASD so finger cymbals should not be introduced until students have had successful experiences with other instruments. Alternately, students can pinch their index fingers and thumbs on the outsides of the elastic. While this hold is easier to obtain, it creates a risk of dropping the instrument if the index finger and thumb do not remain secure. The sounds created by finger cymbals are relatively quiet. In addition, while the sounds continue to ring until the cymbals cease vibrating, they can immediately be muffled by holding the cymbals against the body or by cupping the cymbals in one's hand.

Cluster bells

Cluster bells are a set of three jingle bells, one at the top and one on either side, attached to a plastic handle (see Figure 6.3). The child holds the handle and shakes his or her lower arm to create sounds. Depending on the density of the desired sounds, students may shake a pair of bells, one in each hand. By holding and playing an instrument in each hand, players with ASD have opportunities to develop motor control on both sides of the body and to practice coordination between the two sides of the body

Jingle bells

The sounds of a single jingle bell are enhanced when numerous bells are attached to form groups. Normally, sets of bells are attached to a handle (see Figure 6.3). The child holds the handle, with one or both hands, and shakes his or her lower arms.

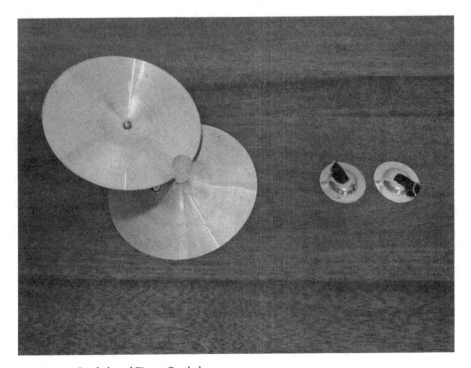

FIGURE 6.2 Cymbals and Finger Cymbals

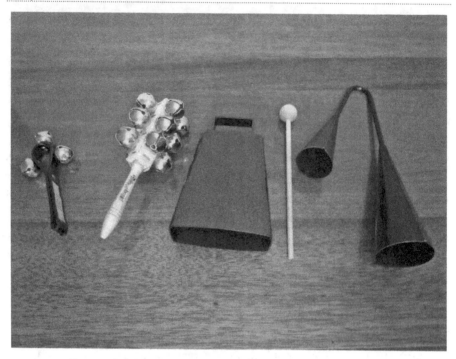

FIGURE 6.3 Cluster Bells, Jingle Bells, Cowbell and Mallet, and Agogo Bells

The number of bells influences the weight of the instrument so, for example, a set of 25 bells is heavier than a set of 12. If a teacher has various sets, the instrument chosen can be matched to the size and strength of the child. As well, the more bells attached to a single handle, the denser the sound produced. Teachers may choose to introduce jingle bells after students with ASD are accustomed to cluster bells as the sounds produced by the latter instrument are more dense than those produced by the former.

Cowbell

Made of metal, cowbells are rectangular-shaped bells with a handle at the top and an open bottom (see Figure 6.3). Traditionally, a clapper attached to the inside of the bell created sounds when the movements of the animal resulted in movements in the bell. The cowbells used as percussion instruments generally do not include clappers. The player grasps the bell by the handle and strikes the body of the instrument with a mallet or a drum stick. The intensity of the sounds produced by the cowbell may cause discomfort to some students with ASD. Teachers may wish to introduce this instrument after students have experience with other instruments that produce metal-like sounds. As well, a student with ASD may first experience this instrument when it is played by another person, so that the student's proximity to the sound may be adjusted based on the student's reactions to the sound.

Agogo bells

Agogo bells are conical-shaped bells that produce sounds reminiscent of cowbells (see Figure 6.3). The classroom variety is generally a set of two bells attached by a narrow u-shaped piece of metal. The bells are different sizes with the sound produced by the larger bell lower than the sound produced by the smaller bell. The player grasps the bells by the strip of metal and holds the instrument in front of him- or herself. The player strikes the bells with a mallet held in the other hand. Similar to the cowbell, the strident sound produced by agogo bells may be difficult for students with ASD to handle.

Triangle

As the name indicates, the triangle is a piece of metal formed in the shape of a triangle and left open at one corner (see Figure 6.4). A loop of string is sometimes used as a holder and some commercial models are attached to small plastic handles. The striker is a small rod of metal. The player holds the triangle and strikes the surface on the side opposite the open corner. Triangles may be purchased in a variety of sizes, giving options for suiting the size of the instrument to the size of the player. I have worked with students with ASD for whom the triangle seems to be one of their favorite instruments. As with finger cymbals, the reverberations created by the triangle may be dampened by placing the instrument against the body or by grabbing the instrument with the free hand.

Cabasa

A cabasa is constructed of a wooden or plastic cylindrical frame with a covering of serrated metal around which a chain of small steel balls is wrapped. The player rests the instrument, chain side down, in the open palm of one hand. Holding the handle in the other hand, the player twists the handle back and forth. This causes the chain of steel balls to scrape against the serrated metal. Students with ASD who have difficulty with small motor movement may find it difficult to play the instrument in this manner. Alternately, sounds may be created by holding the instrument by the handle and shaking it. This less common way to play the instrument creates quieter sounds.

Tambourine

A tambourine consists of a round frame, usually made of wood or plastic, affixed with several pairs of small metal jingles (see Figure 6.5). Traditionally, the term tambourine referred to an instrument with a drumhead. Tambourines for classroom use may be purchased with or without drumheads. The player generally holds the instrument in one hand and shakes the instrument by moving his or her arm. The instrument may also be patted against the body. Alternately, the player can stabilize the

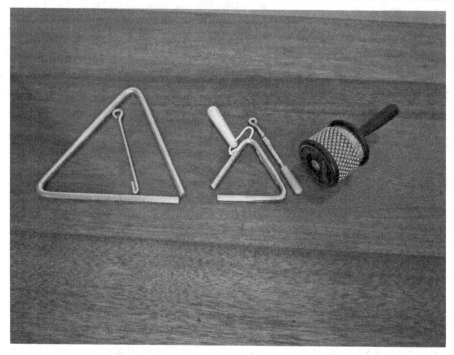

FIGURE 6.4 Triangles and their Beaters, and Cabasa

instrument with one arm or hand and tap the rim of the instrument with the other hand. Tambourines with drumheads may be played by tapping the head with a hand or a mallet. An assortment of sizes allows the teacher to suit the instruments to particular students. A half-moon tambourine is often used by students in schools (see Figure 6.5). This instrument has a rounded side with jingles and a flat side that serves as a handle. In terms of the family of instruments that create metal-like sounds, this is a good starter instrument for students with ASD as the sounds produced are not as strident as those produced by cowbells or the agogo bells and, typically, not as high-pitched as those produced by triangles and finger cymbals.

Skins (hand drum)

There are various types and sizes of drums. A hand drum consists of a narrow circular frame with a drumhead attached to one face (see Figure 6.6). Traditionally, drumheads were made of animal hides; hence their classification as *skins*. Many of the hand drums currently used in elementary-level schools are made of synthetic materials. A hand drum is given its name by the way it is played. Depending on the structure of the instrument, the student holds the drum in one hand, either by grasping the frame, by placing the index finger through a hole on the frame, or by grasping a handle attached to the underside of the instrument. The drum may be

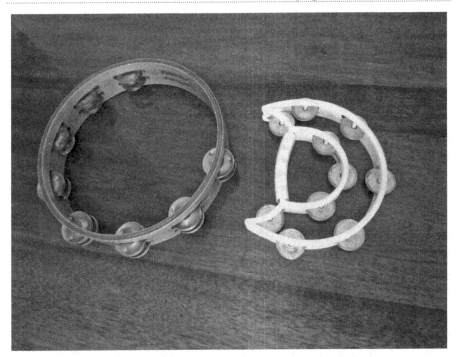

FIGURE 6.5 Tambourine and Half-Moon Tambourine

played with the tips of the fingers or the flat of the hand. Sound effects can be made by sliding the palm or the tips of the fingers across the drumhead. The drum can also be placed on the floor with the head facing up and played with mallets (Berarducci, nd). In my own educational practice I found that drums are a good starting instrument for exploring the beat as it is relatively easy for students with ASD to become accustomed to the sounds produced by this instrument.

Woods

In comparison to metal instruments, the sounds produced by instruments made of wood tend to be relatively easy for students with ASD to accept. The short duration of sounds produced by instruments made of wood may also contribute to students' capacities to work with this family of instruments.

Wood block

A wood block is a rectangular piece of wood with a hollow center (see Figure 6.6). The player balances the woodblock with the fingers of one hand and, using the other hand, strikes the center of the block with a mallet. Students should not rest the woodblock in the palm of their hand as this dampens the sound.

Tick tock block

The tick tock block is a variation of the wood block (see Figure 6.6). It consists of two cylindrically-shaped, hollow objects attached to a handle. The player holds the tick tock block in one hand and strikes the mid-area of the cylinders with a mallet. Since the cylinders are of two different sizes, each produces a different pitch. The instrument gets its name from the idea that, because of the minor third between the pitches of the cylinders, playing one and then the other sounds like a ticking clock.

Sand blocks

Sand blocks come in pairs. They are rectangular blocks with sand paper attached to one side. Small handles made of wood or plastic are attached at the midpoint of the upper side of the blocks (see Figure 6. 6). The student holds these handles and rubs the sandpaper edges across each other to produce scraping sounds. When sand blocks are new, small grains of sand tend to fall from the instruments when they are played. This may be a concern for students with ASD as they may not like the sensation of sand if they feel it on their clothes or skin. As the instrument is used, less and less sand is dislodged as the blocks are scraped together.

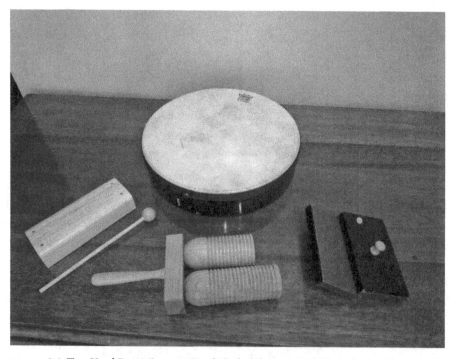

FIGURE 6.6 Top: Hand Drum; Bottom: Wood Block and Beater, Tick Tock Block, and Sand Blocks

Rhythm sticks

Rhythm sticks are made of wood and may be smooth or ribbed (see Figure 6.7). The bright colors of commercially made rhythm sticks (typically green, blue, red, and yellow) tend to appeal to students with ASD. As much as possible, I try to motivate these students by choosing instruments that reflect an individual student's favorite color. Sounds are produced by holding one stick stationary and tapping it with its partner. The ribbed sticks can be rubbed against each other to produce contrasting sounds.

Claves

Claves are a pair of cylindrical sticks made of hardwood (often rosewood). They are approximately 8 inches (20 centimeters) in length and 1 inch (2.5 centimeters) in diameter (see Figure 6.7). The student holds one of the claves with thumb and forefinger grasping the long sides of the instrument. The palm does not make contact with the clave as this dampens the sound. The player grasps the other clave at one end. This becomes the striker that taps the instrument that is held in the other hand. Claves are difficult to play as players need control of small motor muscles to hold the clave with the thumb and fingers and good eye-to-hand coordination to use the striker efficiently. Due to challenges with small muscle movements and hand-eye coordination students on the autism spectrum may have difficulties with these tasks. For demonstrating beat and rhythm, rhythm sticks are a better choice because they are easier to handle and not as fragile.

Guiro

The guiro is from Latin America. It is a hollow instrument with notches around its surface (see Figure 6.7). Sound is produced by scraping a wooden stick across the notches. The instrument has two holes drilled in its bottom. The player holds the instrument by placing thumb and middle finger through the notches. If this is too difficult, the student may grasp the narrow portion at the back of the instrument. If a student needs further support, an assistant may hold the instrument so the student only has to scrape the instrument with the stick, preferably using one hand. The stick may be held with both hands if the student needs to in order to successfully play this instrument.

Sound Effects

Specialized instruments may also be used as sound effects. The items included here are made of metal or wood.

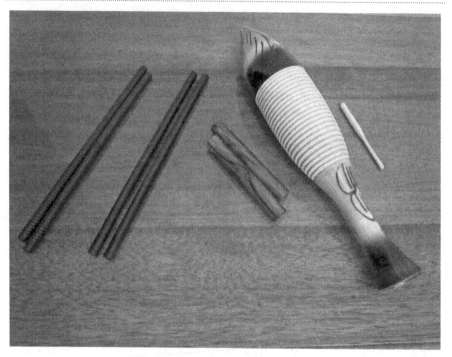

FIGURE 6.7 Rhythm Sticks (Ribbed and Smooth), Claves, and Guiro with Scraping Stick

Wow earth bell

A wow earth bell is a small metal cylinder with a small circular hole drilled toward the bottom (see Figure 6.8). The player grasps the cylinder by the end closest to this hole and strikes the cylinder with a small rubber mallet. The sound is varied by moving the thumb across the hole. Students with ASD may have difficulties accepting the high-pitched sounds produced by this instrument.

Frog guiro

A frog guiro is a frog-shaped instrument with notches along the animal's back (see Figure 6.8). Using the same principle as a standard guiro, the player scrapes a stick across the notches to create sounds reflective of a croaking frog. This instrument is well suited to those students with ASD who are visual learners, as the shape of the instrument is strongly-related to the sound it produces.

Owl whistle

An owl whistle is, as its name suggests, a whistle in the shape of an owl (see Figure 6.8). The player produces the sounds of a hooting owl by blowing through a hole at a back of the owl's head. To avoid passing germs from one student to the next, in my classes the owl whistle is only played by the teacher. As with the frog guiro, there is a close association of the shape of the instrument and the sound it produces, which can help those students with ASD who are visual learners to identify this instrument.

Train whistle

Train whistles manufactured for use with and by young students are short lengths of square-sectioned wood with, usually, four holes drilled lengthwise (see Figure 6.8). The player grasps the instrument and blows through the holes at the top. In contrast to the sounds produced by trains, this whistle creates a relatively quiet and breathy sound. I often use this instrument in improvisational storytelling with students on the autism spectrum.

HOW INSTRUMENTS ARE PLAYED

Instruments are also categorized by how they are played by students in school activities: blowing, scraping, shaking, and striking (see Table 6.2).

Even though the hand drum may be played by scraping one's hand across its surface, it is categorized with instruments that players strike, as this is the way the hand drum is played most often by students in schools. Instruments that are often played in more than one way are listed twice. For example, it is equally possible to strike or

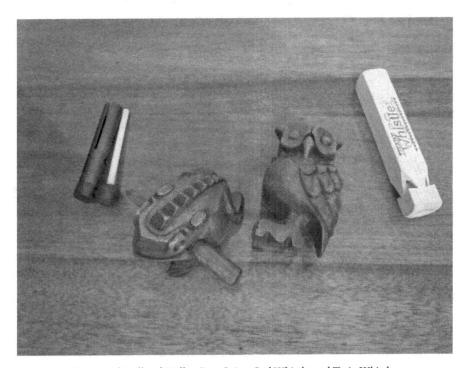

FIGURE 6.8 Wow Earth Bell and Mallet, Frog Guiro, Owl Whistle, and Train Whistle

TABLE 6.2

How Instruments are Played

striking	shaking	scraping	blowing
wood block	egg shakers	rhythm sticks	owl whistle
tick tock block	chikitas	sand blocks	train whistle
triangle	maracas	guiro	
cowbell	cluster bells	cabasa	
agogo bells	jingle bells		
wow earth bell	tambourine		
rhythm sticks			
claves			
finger cymbals			
drum			
tambourine			

scrape rhythm sticks; the tambourine is played both by shaking and striking. The order of the instruments is derived from the specifics of their construction and how they are played. For example, egg shakers, chikitas, and maracas are grouped together because they are similar in construction and create similar sounds. Cluster bells and jingle bells use the same bells in their construction. Instruments that players strike are grouped according to what they are struck with. Instruments played with mallets are grouped at the top of this column; instruments with which players strike each member of a pair together are in the middle; instruments that players strike (tap) with their hands are at the bottom.

EASE OF PERFORMANCE

Many students on the autism spectrum have difficulties coordinating body movements (Morin & Reid, 1985; Staples & Reid, 2010) and experience challenges with eye-hand coordination (Dowd, McGinley, Taffe, & Rinehart, 2012). They may also have difficulties estimating the amount of physical energy needed to complete psychomotor tasks. Many of these students use more force than is necessary when playing musical instruments, and may need reminders to play more gently (describing the force) or more quietly (describing the volume of the sound produced). For these reasons, the physical demands of the instruments must be balanced with the physical challenges of the students so that the instruments chosen suit each student's level of functioning. This does not imply that students are not encouraged to stretch their expertise beyond the current levels. Rather, instruments are chosen carefully, beginning with those that place fewer demands on motor skills and eye-hand coordination. After students have successful experiences with the instruments that are easiest to play, they are guided toward those that are more difficult. While there is no definitive progression of non-pitched percussion instruments for students with ASD, Table 6.3 addresses this need, taking into account both the physical requirements for playing technique and the physical challenges of students with ASD.

Given that students on the spectrum vary in many ways, it is not possible to devise a list that will predict the sequence of percussion performance for all individuals. Rather, this listing of instruments is a guide. Teachers use professional judgment in making performance decisions for their students, keeping in mind that students with ASD may need more practice to develop the skills to play these instruments than their typically developing peers.

TABLE 6.3

Ease of Performance Listed from
Easiest to Most Difficult to Play

Instrument
hand drum
tambourine
chikitas
jingle bells
maracas
egg shakers
cluster bells
rhythm sticks
woodblock
tick tock block
cowbell
agogo bells
triangle
finger cymbals
sand blocks
guiro
cabasa
cymbals
claves

In general, the hand drum is a viable beginning instrument for many students. Hand drums are available in a variety of sizes (e.g., 6, 8, 10, and 12 inches [15, 20, 25, and 30 centimeters]). This variety provides teachers with options in choosing an instrument that suits the size of the child. While eye-hand coordination is needed for the hand to make contact with the drumhead, the size of the drum eases this requirement. If the child has difficulty coordinating hand movements, an assistant may hold the drum, leaving the child with the sole task of striking the drum. The tambourine requires similar technique to the drum. This is especially the case when the tambourine has a drumhead. If not, the player must adjust his or her hand to strike on the rim of the instrument. While it is important for students to eventually use both hands in playing instruments, an assistant may hold drums or tambourines if a student finds it difficult to engage both hands when playing instruments. Alternately, the drum or tambourine may be attached to a stand.

Instruments that students hold and shake include chikitas, jingle bells, maracas, egg shakers, and cluster bells. The eye-hand coordination required when playing these instruments is minimal when compared to many of the other instruments. Players are expected to hold and shake the instruments but do not need to strike them with a mallet using their free hands. Coordinated movements are needed, however, to synchronize the instruments so that both hands shake the instruments at the same time or so the sounds alternate from one instrument to its partner. If a student finds it difficult to engage both hands simultaneously, the student may begin by holding a single shaker in the hand of his or her choice. Chikitas and cluster bells are smaller and lighter in weight and are therefore easier to play than maracas and jingle bells. From a practical standpoint, chikitas and cluster bells are better starter instruments as they can withstand some rough treatment, such as unintentional drops. They are relatively inexpensive so are easier to replace than some of the other instruments. The egg shaker is the most difficult to play in this group as it seems that many students find it easier to grasp handles than cup objects in the palms of their hands.

Rhythm sticks are fundamental to classroom music. Due to their relatively low cost (in comparison to other musical instruments), it may be possible to have a class set so that all students can play rhythm sticks at the same time. Sounds are created when the player holds one stick stationary and taps the other against its partner. Using this technique when playing rhythm sticks takes careful modeling on the part of teachers and practice from the students. Some individuals tend to move both sticks towards each other until they make contact. This requires greater attention to hand-eye coordination and often results in inaccurate performances as the students have less control over when the sticks make contact. Claves look similar to rhythm sticks, but the technique differs, with the claves being more difficult to play.

Woodblock, tick tock block, cowbell, agogo bells, and triangle are grouped together because they all require the player to strike the instrument with a mallet (or a striker [triangle]). Finger cymbals are included in this group because the weight and material pose challenges similar to those involved in playing the triangle. Instruments played with a mallet pose challenges for eye-hand coordination as students must anticipate where to strike the mallet on the instrument. As well, students must estimate the force needed to create appropriate tones.

The triangle and finger cymbals have their own set of challenges. As with the finger cymbals, many of the smaller triangles (e.g., 4 inches [10 centimeters] or 7 inches [18 centimeters]) are light in weight. Little effort is needed to create the desired sound by gently tapping the instrument. If too much effort is used the instruments may move erratically, making it difficult to coordinate movements if the student is required to play the instrument a second time in short succession. As well, triangles and finger cymbals create distractions for students with ASD who may focus on the reflections created by the instruments' surfaces and thereby disengage from the class.

Sand blocks, guiro, and cabasa require the player to perform sideways motions. It is difficult to judge which of these instruments is the easiest to play. The sand block relies on larger muscle motions. However, it requires that players coordinate back and forth movements of both hands and arms. When playing the guiro the student needs fine motor skills to grasp a small stick while, at the same time, hold the instrument with the other hand. The cabasa requires that one hand is stationary while the other hand grasps the handle. As well, students must accept the tactile stimulation of the weight of the instrument in their palm as the metal balls scrape across the serrated metal background. Cymbals differ from the above instruments in terms of how they are played, but they pose similar challenges in motor control as one cymbal is held stationary while large motor muscles are engaged in the other arm so that the second cymbal makes contact with its partner. These instruments should be introduced after students have gained some facility with instruments that are easier to play.

General Guidelines for Teachers

- Use only a few instruments at a time. This is especially the case when first introducing the instruments as students with ASD might find a large array of unfamiliar objects visually overwhelming. The cacophony of sounds produced by a large number of unfamiliar instruments may also be difficult to handle.
- Use all of the instruments that are within the students' fields of vision to avoid disappointment if some instruments are not used (Birkenshaw-Fleming,

1993). This will also avoid difficulties if some students are unable to accept that the class is finished when all of the materials have not been used.

- If unsure of which instruments you will use, arrange them so they can be presented efficiently but that students are not aware of their presence. For example, instruments may be placed in boxes or on shelves hidden under sheets. This will help students to focus on current tasks without being distracted by the presence of the instruments and students will not be disappointed or upset if some instruments are not used.

- Always model respect for the instruments and ensure that students handle the instruments with care (Bruscia, 1987). Some instruments, such as rhythm sticks, can be played vigorously with a low likelihood of damage. This makes them good beginning instruments. In contrast, the more delicate rosewood claves might crack if dropped accidentally. This more fragile instrument is used after students have gained some competency in holding and playing classroom percussion instruments.

- Pay particular attention to the students' reactions to these sounds. Some students on the autism spectrum might be particularly sensitive to some of the timbres (e.g., the loud clanking sounds of a cowbell). If the sounds of particular instruments cause distress, teachers may choose to avoid those instruments until students have had time to gain familiarity with the timbres produced by instruments that do not inflict such disturbance.

- Given the difficulties experienced in balance (Vernazza-Martin et al., 2005) and coordination (Morin & Reid, 1985; Staples & Reid, 2010), it is recommended that students sit on the floor, especially when first learning how to hold and play musical instruments.

- Suit the instruments to each student's motor skills. Consider, for example, a child with difficulties in eye/hand coordination. When playing rhythm sticks the child grasps the sticks with both hands and has a large area to strike when producing the required sounds. In comparison, finger cymbals are held by the thumbs and index fingers and require a small movement of one hand to strike the side of one cymbal with its partner. For these reasons, rhythm sticks present fewer obstacles for a child at an early point in his or her motor development.

- Provide opportunities for students to play a variety of instruments as well as opportunities for them to play their favorite instruments.

- Adjust the pace of the class, providing extra time to individuals who need more time to respond.

- Be attentive to the effort or energy used to play the instruments. If a child plays too harshly, verbal reminders to play more gently may be helpful. Create a game by asking students to adjust their performance to different levels of dynamics. Begin with *forte* (loud), as this reflects the dynamic level of playing too harshly. Gradually move to *mezzo forte* (moderately loud), *mezzo piano* (moderately quiet), and *piano* (quiet). If this approach is not successful, try giving the child a different instrument. If the child continues to play too harshly it may be necessary to move to another activity (Borczon, 2004).

- Discourage the students' use of classroom percussion instruments for self-stimulation (e.g., spinning triangles by light sources) as this behavior inhibits opportunities for joint attention. Sometimes self-stimulation may be interrupted by motivating the student to take part in classroom activities. For example, if a student is using a triangle for self-stimulation, an adult might gain the student's attention by playing an instrument with a different timbre, such as rhythm sticks. If the student is engrossed in playing the triangle, the teacher might gain the student's attention by imitating the rhythmic patterns the student is producing (see Instrumental Conversations Using Rhythm Sticks later in this chapter).

- If these strategies are unsuccessful it may be necessary to put the instruments away and move to another activity.

- Using mallets adds additional requirements to instrument playing. Students must hold the instrument in one hand, grip the mallet in the other hand, activate the muscle control needed to strike the instrument with the appropriate amount of force, and coordinate eye and hand movements to ensure that the mallet strikes the instrument in the proper place. The introduction of mallets may begin with providing the student opportunities to experiment with an instrument that is played with a mallet, for example, a wood block:

- Hand the mallet to the student and allow him or her to explore how the object feels and how it is shaped.

- Dissuade the student from dropping or throwing the mallet so that this activity does not replace interest in its use as a musical instrument (Streeter, 1993). It is also important to discourage dropping or throwing the mallet so that this act does not become a part of the student's routine for playing the instrument.

- Hand-over-hand assistance may be needed. At first, the assistant may need to hold his or her hand over the student's grip (Streeter, 1993). As the child is able to grasp the mallet, the assistant's hand may move further up the wrist (Nordoff & Robbins, 2007).

- Be careful that the assistant supports the student and encourages the student's attempts to play the instrument (Streeter, 1993). While the assistant may gently guide the student to play the beat (Nordoff & Robbins, 2007), the assistant should not impose musical patterns on the student (Streeter, 1993) as the student may lose interest if the student feels he or she is not managing the situation and/or is unable to keep up with his or her peers.

- Maintain realistic expectations. Students may not be able to coordinate the movements needed to play instruments with mallets until provided with practice over several class sessions (Streeter, 1993).

Moving on from free exploration, students acquire the ability to play instruments in the intended manner(s) and to follow the teacher's directions for engaging in structured activities. Using proper playing techniques and following the teacher's directions requires that teachers, instructional assistants, and typically developing peers all model appropriate behaviors. While the ultimate goal is for students on the autism spectrum to play the instruments in traditionally correct ways, views of acceptable playing technique must be sensitive to the needs and proclivities of all learners.

While accommodating individual differences, it is important that musical instruments are treated with respect. It is not appropriate for cowbells and maracas to be thrown on the floor when an activity is finished; nor is it acceptable for a student to release frustrations by hitting caregivers or peers with rhythm sticks or woodblocks. These are aspects of general decorum that must be reinforced. Beyond that though, it is more important for students on the autism spectrum to be involved in classroom activities than it is for these students to play musical instruments with *perfect* technique.

Students' Initial Experiences

Percussion instruments are introduced gradually, perhaps only one or two at a time, with multiple opportunities for students to gain comfort with holding and playing these instruments before more are introduced. For this reason, the initial experience with instruments is not a one-time occurrence. Rather, procedures for initial experimentation and performance occur repeatedly as new instruments are added to the students' repertoire.

In general, it is unrealistic to assume that students on the autism spectrum will respond positively to percussion instruments as soon they are introduced. Some students need time to accept and adjust to changes in the environment as these instruments appear. The behaviors that teachers and other caregivers might observe from their students (ignore, engage, involve, commit) resemble those described in Chapter 4 as responses to the introduction of the scarf game (see pages 112 to 113).

SENSORY STIMULATION

Playing instruments is a multi-dimensional sensory experience, involving simultaneous aural, visual, tactile, and motor processing. This sensory stimulation comprises the following elements:

Aural: The student hears the instrument, discerns where the sound originates, and perceives the timbre.

Visual: The child identifies the instrument by its shape and identifies what the instrument is made of.

Tactile: The child identifies what the instrument is made of, accepts the tactile sensations of holding the instrument, and interprets the tactile sensations of the vibrations created when sounds are produced.

Motor: The child initiates and maintains movements needed to hold the instrument, enacts movements to play the instrument in the appropriate manner, and gauges the energy or force needed to produce the appropriate sounds.

EXPLORATION

The teacher sits on the floor or on a low chair or stool that allows interaction with the students at the same physical level (e.g., eye-to-eye and hand-to-hand). The teacher introduces each instrument by sharing basic background information:

- The instrument's name (e.g., drum)
- What the instrument is made of (e.g., skin)
- How it is played (e.g., hold the instrument by the handle and strike the edges of the skin with the tips of the fingers or the flat of the hand).

After providing basic background information, the teacher plays the instrument so students have the opportunity to hear the sounds produced. The teacher gives students opportunities for free exploration. When working with students on the autism spectrum, this may require patience and prodding over time. The following descriptions outline actions that teachers might implement when encouraging engagement from these students. This is not a step-by-step set of procedures. Rather, these descriptions highlight some of the situations teachers might encounter with their students and provide advice on how they could proceed.

- Place the instrument in front of a student.
- Encourage the student to pick it up. If the student hesitates, the teacher can point to the instrument while saying its name and, using body language, encourage the student to pick it up.
- The teacher plays the instrument and waits, watching what the student does. If the student picks up the instrument or in some way taps or strikes it so that sound emits, this action is rewarded by verbal responses such as 'good playing' accompanied by hand claps to signal a positive reaction. Teachers should use whatever procedures are in place to reward particular students.
- If the student does not pick up the instrument, the teacher might place it in one of the student's hands. If this does not result in a reaction from the student, the teacher could play the instrument or, using a hand over hand technique, place the student's hand on the instrument so that it produces a sound. Repetition of this procedure might help the student realize that he or she is able to play the instrument (adapted from Nordoff & Robbins, 2007).
- Allow free time for the student to explore the instrument, turning it over in his or her hands to see it from all sides and striking or shaking it to produce a variety of sounds. Experimentation includes the production of sounds in nonconventional ways, such as shaking a cabasa as if it were a maraca, provided that doing so does not damage the instrument (Alvin, 1991).
- Present another instrument or move to another activity if the student is using the instrument for self-stimulation, for instance by repeatedly spinning a rhythm stick on the floor.

If the teacher is working with small groups of students, the sharing of one instrument across class members may be feasible. If a teacher is working with a large class comprised of both students with ASD and their typically developing peers, multiple instruments may be passed around the class. This increases the probability that all students (or most) will be able to handle the object during the class and facilitates classroom management by keeping the students involved in classroom activities. For example, if the activity or goal is introducing the hand drum, the teacher passes three or four drums to students sitting in different areas of the circle so that more than one student is able to experiment with a drum at the same time. This is not always feasible as the cost of instruments may prohibit ownership of multiple items.

The way instruments are handled also depends on the temperaments of individual students and how these individuals collaborate as a group. Ideally, teachers envision groups of students in which all individuals are content to sit in the circle and wait their turn. This does not reflect the reality of many teachers' lives. For this reason, individual teachers use professional judgment in deciding how to plan the introduction of instruments in their own classrooms

Teachers experiment with the order in which they introduce non-pitched percussion instruments to determine whether there is a sequence that works better for their program and with their students. I begin with the hand drum. This decision comes from the practicalities of my own teaching situation. First, I own sufficient drums so that each student has his or her own instrument for ensemble work; second, the drum can comfortably sit in a student's lap or can easily be held by the handle or on the side (depending on the make and/or model); third, holding the drum with one hand, the child can tap the drum with the other hand, thereby avoiding the coordination of both hands for proper tone production; fourth, the drum is open to experimentation as different sounds may be produced by tapping the drum with the fingers, the flat of the hand, or by sliding the palm across its surface; fifth, the drum provides a tactile experience as it is the touch from the player that creates the sound: sixth, drums can be purchased in several sizes, thereby allowing some personalization of the instrument in relation to the size of the player. After students are familiar with hand drums, I introduce rhythm sticks.. Rhythm sticks are similar to the hand drum in that both instruments are played by striking. Unlike the hand drum, when playing rhythm sticks the player holds one stick in each hand and strikes one stick with the other. This requires increased eye-hand coordination and hand–to-hand coordination.

Next, I introduce instruments that are shaken. Depending on the student's readiness, the student can play one instrument in the hand of his or her choice. Doing so avoids the challenge of coordinating movements on the left and right side of the body. Next are instruments played with mallets such as cowbell, wood block, and tick tock block. These instruments rely on the student's ability to control the effort or force needed to strike the object with the mallet and also on the student's attention to eye-hand coordination.

I include additional instruments based on the interest and readiness of the students. An increasing variety of instruments, such as cabasa, finger cymbals, guiro, and triangle can be introduced to further explore timbre when creating instrumental accompaniments for picture books and personal stories as described later in this chapter.

EDUCATIONAL INTERVENTIONS

Educational interventions include activities in which the whole class plays instruments, activities in which small groups of students play instruments, and activities in which individual students play instruments one at a time. As a class moves from one activity to the next, students listen to the directions provided by the teacher, understand the meaning, and demonstrate this understanding by following through with the requested behaviors. When using a small number of instruments, clear directions for social interaction and sharing are effective. For example, the teacher might say, "Laura, your turn is finished. Please hand the agogo bells to Brent." Laura might follow these directions by handing the instrument to Brent. When working with students who are not accustomed to following directions, establishing this routine takes time and patience. In addition, teachers and instructional assistants are attentive to students' requests where appropriate (see text box 6.1).

The educational interventions included in this chapter are arranged in two groups: experiences in which students listen to and demonstrate understanding of specific properties in what they hear, and activities where students play musical instruments.

Aural acuity

Aural acuity refers to the students' understanding of instruments' sounds. As described above, the classroom percussion instruments may be categorized according to four families based on the materials used to produce the sounds: gourds, metals, skins, and woods. Classroom activities develop the students' ability to identify instruments' sounds by the family to which the instrument belongs and to identify a particular instrument by its sound.

Instrument family identification

The teacher sets up a situation in which students can hear an instrument but do not see it. Their task is to identify the family to which the instrument belongs based on the sounds produced. If choosing from four families of instruments is overwhelming,

---

TEXT BOX 6.1
CLASSROOM VIGNETTE

Marissa, a student with ASD, is reluctant to join her peers in movement activities. She indicates her enjoyment by smiling and laughing while she watches the other children. One day she wants to communicate but cannot find the words. When asked what she wants, she mimes playing a musical instrument. After showing her a wood block and a tick tock block, the teacher held up a triangle. This was the instrument Marissa wanted. She happily accompanied the students' movements with her triangle. This did not interrupt the activities of the rest of the class so this became her means of involvement on that particular day.

students could begin by choosing between two instrument families (e.g., metals or woods) with possible choices expanded to all four families of instruments after students gain familiarity with this task.

The way that students indicate their responses may take many forms, depending on the set-up of the classroom and the number of students in the class. For example:

- Visuals of instruments and their families are arranged on the walls. Students point to the visuals to indicate the family of the instrument they hear.
- Each child has a set of four cards with visuals representing a different family of instruments on each card. Each child selects the card that illustrates the family of the instrument. Students can complete this task while working with partners.

After the students indicate their choices, the leader reveals the instrument and plays it again. In preparation for subsequent activities, the leader asks a student to name the instrument. If no one remembers the name, the teacher provides this information.

Specific instrument identification

After students are adept at categorizing instrument timbres by their families, they are ready to engage in the similar, but more demanding, task of identifying instruments by the sounds they produce. This activity may take several forms, including the following:

- Two individuals (instructional assistants or students) stand at the front of the class. They each hold a different instrument. The teacher (or designate) plays an instrument hidden from view and the students choose what they hear by pointing to the person holding that instrument.
- The students view pictures of assorted instruments posted on the walls and point to the instrument they hear.
- Each child has a set of small cards with photos or illustrations of the instruments and chooses the card corresponding to the instrument heard. Students can complete this task while working with partners.

The number of cards and characteristics of the instruments illustrated on the cards is adjusted as students gain competence with this task. Choices may begin with two instruments with dissimilar timbres, such as a cowbell and a triangle. If students are able to discriminate between the sounds created by these instruments, they might be asked to discriminate between two instruments with similar sounds, such as jingle bells and cluster bells or wood block and tick tock block. As a student progresses, the number of choices increases.

PLAYING INSTRUMENTS
Accompanying songs

Through my experiences as a music teacher I have observed that, in general, students with ASD readily tap the beat in response to songs and singing. Adding non-pitched percussion instruments is a next step in extending these experiences. Playing percussion instruments motivates students toward active participation in making music. This is especially the case for students on the autism spectrum who may be unable to sing or who may have limited verbal abilities.

The number of instrumentalists depends on the size of the class, the type of instruments used, and the sounds produced. When possible, sufficient numbers of rhythm sticks, jingle bells, and chikitas allow all students to play these instruments at the same time. Depending on class size, purchase of this number of instruments may take place over a span of several years, beginning with rhythm sticks and with jingle bells or chikitas added next, depending on the way particular teachers decide to use the instruments. It is desirable to have sufficient drums so that each child can play or that students can work in pairs or trios, with each group sharing a drum. A teacher may want to have an assortment of triangles and tambourines so that multiple students may play these instruments at the same time. As well, if the teacher has multiple items of different sizes, the instrument can be suited to the size of the student. For the remaining exercises profiled here, only one or two of each is needed.

Teachers need to be aware that the sounds produced by groups of instruments, and especially groups of instruments with disparate sounds, may be overwhelming for some students on the autism spectrum. Teachers observe their students carefully for any outward signs of distress such as placing their hands over their ears, jumping up and down, flapping hands, or rocking. In assessing how to help students, it is necessary to take into account the timbres produced by the instruments. The sounds produced when all students play rhythm sticks or drums may not bother a student with ASD as the sounds produced by these instruments are relatively low in pitch and do not continue to ring out once the instrument has been played. On the other hand, the sounds produced by several triangles or pairs of finger cymbals may be difficult to adjust to as the sounds are relatively high and continue to ring once the instruments have been struck. As well, instruments such as cowbells and agogo bells are relatively loud when compared to the other percussion instruments profiled here. These considerations may guide instrument choices as teachers create a comfortable learning environment for all students.

Beat

Performing the beat may begin with students showing the beat in songs by clapping their hands, patting their laps, stamping their feet or performing other physical movements that reflect the beat. This perception of the beat is then transferred to instruments.

Drums and rhythm sticks are excellent choices for introductory activities in which students play the beat on instruments to accompany songs. The song *This Old Man* makes reference to a drum in the first verse, creating a logical fit for students to play drums while singing the song. As students are better able to coordinate their movements with the beat, wood blocks and jingle bells may be added to this list of choices. Students need a good sense of timing to coordinate sounds produced by maracas (chikitas) or cabasa to accompany the beat when singing songs. These instruments are used to accompany singing after students have gained proficiency in demonstrating the beat on other instruments. Keeping in mind the character of the songs, the cabasa may be a suitable instrument for playing the beat while singing the song *Fall is on Its Way* because the sound of the instrument helps create the image of the crunching sounds made by dried leaves.

Some instruments, such as triangles and finger cymbals, are not well suited to playing the beat because students may need time to stabilize the instrument and readjust their eye-hand coordination each time they play these instruments. If the sounds produced by these instruments create the desired imagery for a given piece, rather than playing the beat the students could play their instruments at the beginning of phrases. This technique is often found in materials based around the Orff approach for music education (Steen, 1992).

Playing every beat to accompany songs may be easier than using instruments at the beginning of phrases or to accompany particular words. When students play every beat they do not need to be concerned about which beats to play. If playing at the beginning of phrases, the students must be aware of the sequence of sounds and silences and play their instruments only at the appropriate time. This may be especially difficult for those students who find it difficult to perform motor sequences (Hardy & LaGasse, 2013; Hughes, 1996; Rinehart, Bradshaw, Brereton, & Tonge, 2001; Todd, 2012). This does not imply that these students are not able to perform activities with musical instruments that require them to sequence movements according to patterns in music. Rather, teachers need to be aware that students on the autism spectrum may need more time and practice to accomplish these tasks than their typically developing peers. Students might benefit from visual support, such as a helper (instructional assistant or peer) who through hand movements indicates when to play the instrument. Physical assistance, such as hand-over-hand guidance, might also be helpful. These supports should be removed as soon as students are able to perform independently.

Expression

Playing instruments at appropriate dynamic levels adds another level of complexity to playing instruments as students must understand the meanings of the words used to describe dynamics (such as loud and quiet) and judge the force used to play the instruments that results in the appropriate sounds. In choosing appropriate instrumentation, it is necessary to take the characteristics of the songs into account. These characteristics may be intrinsic to the songs or may be revealed in contexts derived by the teacher or the students.

Many times the dynamics are intrinsic characteristics of songs. Lullabies, such as *Hush Little Baby and Sleep, Baby, Sleep* are a viable starting place for highlighting tempo and dynamics when playing instruments as, given that the purpose of lullabies is to sooth a baby or small child, it makes sense to sing them quietly and with a moderately slow tempo.

As with singing, teachers create contexts for guiding expressive decisions when playing instruments. Students begin by playing instruments to contrast fast and slow or quiet and loud. After they are able to complete this task, they may move to comparisons that involve dynamics *and* tempo. In so doing, students become aware of four basic pairings: quiet and slow, quiet and fast, loud and slow, and loud and fast. I illustrate scenarios to guide expressive decisions with the song *Row, Row, Row Your Boat*.

QUIET OR LOUD. The teacher might introduce an explanation of loud or quiet with an explanation such as: "We are playing the beat on our drums while we sing *Row, Row, Row Your Boat*. We have two choices, quiet or loud. How would we play so that the dynamics of our playing show our boat floating along in calm waters?" The students might respond with "quietly." Students then sing the song and play their drums quietly. The teacher might then ask a question to create a contrast: "How would we play our dynamics if we were rowing our boat in a storm?" The students might respond with "loudly." The students then sing and play their drums loudly.

FAST OR SLOW. The teacher might introduce fast or slow with an explanation such as: "We are playing the beat on our drums while we sing *Row, Row, Row Your Boat*. We have two choices, fast or slow. How would we play so that the tempo of our playing show that a calm breeze is pushing our boat along in the water?" The students might respond with "slowly." The teacher then sets a slow tempo and the students play their drums. The teacher might then ask a question to create a contrast: "How would we play so the tempo shows the boat in a strong wind?" The students might respond with "fast." The teacher then sets a faster tempo and students play their drums.

QUIET AND SLOW OR QUIET AND FAST. The teacher might introduce quiet and slow or quiet and fast with an explanation such as: "We are playing the beat on our drums while we sing *Row, Row, Row Your Boat*. We have two choices, quiet and slow or quiet and fast. How would our dynamics and tempo show that we are resting in our boat?" The students might respond with "quiet and slow." The teacher then sets a slow tempo; the students play their drums quietly. The teacher might continue by asking "How would our dynamics and tempo show that the people in the boat are late for bedtime and must head for home without waking anyone up?" The students might respond with "quiet and fast." The teacher then sets a fast tempo and the students play their drums quietly.

LOUD AND SLOW OR LOUD AND FAST. The teacher might introduce loud and slow or loud and fast with an explanation such as: "We are playing the beat on our drums while we sing *Row, Row, Row Your Boat*. We have two choices, loud and slow or loud and fast. How might we play so that our dynamics and tempo to show that we are dragging the boat through mud?" The students might respond with "loud and slow." The teacher then sets a slow tempo and the students play their drums loudly. The teacher might continue by asking? "How might we play so our dynamics and tempo show that we are late getting home for supper?" The students might respond with "loud and fast." The teacher then sets a fast tempo; the students play their drums loudly.

Experimenting with Sounds

Students are often introduced to percussion instruments through activities in which they explore and experiment with ways to produce sounds with these instruments. Activities are shared in three separate, but related areas: creating sounds by following the conductor, creating sounds to accompany stories, and creating instrumental conversations.

CREATING SOUNDS BY FOLLOWING THE CONDUCTOR

Each child has a percussion instrument. The choice of instrument depends on the context. The students could all play the same instruments such as drums, rhythm sticks, chikitas, or jingle bells. The students could all play instruments from the same family such as metals or woods. The students could be divided into two groups with one group playing instruments that produce metal sounds and the other group playing instruments that produce wood sounds. The leader conducts the group and the students play their instruments in response to these directions.

For example, the teacher, alone or in collaboration with the students, might devise hand signals that represent the tempo and dynamics with which students are directed to play, such as:

Quiet and slow: small hand movements performed slowly
Quiet and fast: small hand movements performed quickly
Loud and slow: large arm motions performed slowly
Loud and fast: large arm motions performed quickly

The leader performs the movements and the students play their instruments in ways that reflect the tempo and dynamics that are indicated by the movements.

After students are able to follow these directions, new movements could be added, indicating new ways of performance, such as:

Gradually getting louder (*crescendo*): small arm movements that gradually become large arm movements;
Gradually getting quieter (*decrescendo*): large arm movements that gradually become small hand movements.
Gradually getting faster (accelerando): slow arm movements that gradually become fast arm movements.
Gradually getting slower (rallentando): fast arm movements that gradually become slow arm movements.

As with quiet and loud, motions representing *crescendo* and *decrescendo* may be performed slowly or quickly. Teachers are reminded that students on the autism spectrum have difficulties performing gestures they view as meaningless (Smith & Bryson, 2007; Vanvuchelen, Roeyers, & De Weerdt, 2007; Vivanti, Nadig, Ozonoff, & Rogers, 2008; Williams, Whiten, & Singh, 2004). Use of these gestures to represent tempo and dynamics in music needs to be explained carefully to students, along with aural examples of each, so they understand the meaning of the gestures before engaging in the activity.

Instead of using arm signals to represent tempo and dynamics, the teacher could place the directions on a board or screen and point to specific directions to indicate how the students should perform. Depending on the age and experience of the students the descriptions above could be used. Students could also be asked to interpret the Italian terms often used in music to represent tempo and dynamics. For example:

Quiet and slow: *piano* and *largo*
Quiet and fast: *piano* and *presto*
Loud and slow: *forte* and *largo*
Loud and fast: *forte* and *presto*
Gradually getting quieter: *decrescendo*
Gradually getting louder: *crescendo*
Gradually getting faster: *accelerando*
Gradually getting slower: *rallentando*

After students are familiar with the directions, peers could be chosen to lead the class.

If the sound produced by the whole class is too loud and overwhelming for some of the students, smaller groups of students could take turns performing. If all of the students play the same type of instrument (e.g., all playing rhythm sticks), smaller groups of students could be identified based on their placement in the room (e.g., students in the front row). If they are playing different instruments, the smaller groups chosen to play could be identified by instruments (e.g., students with wood-blocks). Smaller groups of instruments could also be identified by families (e.g., students with instruments that produce metal sounds). This activity is especially beneficial for students on the autism spectrum because, along with gaining practice in playing instruments, they have opportunities to follow directions and wait for their turn to play.

CREATING SOUNDS TO ACCOMPANY STORIES
Picture books

Percussion instruments might also be used to enhance the words in picture books. I will discuss two examples: the pairing of *The quiet book* (Underwood & Liwska, 2010) and *The loud book* (Underwood & Liwska, 2011), and the book *Blue sky* (Wood, 2012).

The Quiet Book and The Loud Book

With illustrations of animals engaging in the activities described in the text these books appeal to young students. Each illustration includes a short description of a quiet activity such as not scaring the robin (*The quiet book,* illustration 3) or a loud activity such as the ringing of an alarm clock (*The loud book,* illustration 1).

The following steps outline suggested procedures for using these books as an impetus for students to create quiet and loud sounds with percussion instruments.

To introduce *The quiet book*:

- the teacher reads entries from the book. (e.g., *First one awake*, illustration 1).
- the teacher plays a hand drum quietly after reading each sentence.
- the teacher reads the book and the students play instruments quietly after the teacher reads each sentence. The teacher uses a visual signal (such as a conductor's cut off) to indicate when the students should quit playing their instruments.

After students have sufficient opportunities to respond to the statements in this book by playing their instruments quietly, *The loud book* is introduced using the same steps outlined above.

Teachers adjust the activity in response to the reactions and interest of the students. It is not necessary to read the whole book at any one time as the statements about loud or quiet stand alone. The teacher may continue or terminate the activity whenever students' behaviors indicate that it is time to move to another activity.

The recommendation to introduce *The quiet book* first is based on my experiences working with students on the autism spectrum. Many of these students experience difficulties estimating the amount of force needed to complete motor tasks. When playing instruments they often use more force than necessary and must often be reminded to play *quietly*. If this verbal request does not bring about the desired response, they may be asked to play more *gently*. This order of introduction may avoid any problems that arise if students become accustomed to using the force needed to play loudly and must then adjust this force to create quiet sounds. If teachers find that students are unable to play quietly they may introduce this activity with *The loud book*. On the other hand, they may postpone this activity until students have had sufficient experience and practice with the instruments to be able to exert some control over the dynamic levels they create when playing percussion instruments.

After students are able to follow directions for creating quiet sounds and loud sounds to accompany *The quiet book* or *The loud book*, a version of this activity may be implemented using both books:

- The students are divided into two groups, a loud group and a quiet group.
- The teacher reads a sentence from *The quiet book* and the students in the quiet group create the corresponding sounds on their instruments.

- The teacher reads a sentence from *The loud book* and the students in the loud group create corresponding sounds on their instruments.

The back and forth between quiet and loud continues until the students' interest and/or motivation wanes. If possible, students choose the loud group or the quiet group because, by making choices, they gain a sense of control within the school environment.

Sometimes students, and even adults, assume that loud sounds are fast and quiet sounds are slow. Teachers can use the images in these books to challenge this misconception by asking students to create accompaniments that are loud and slow or accompaniments that are quiet and fast. Activities derived from these books can be related to the activity in which students create sounds by following the conductor. Combining ideas from both activities, a teacher could read a sentence from *The quiet book* or *The loud book* and point to the words to show students how to play the accompaniment. Alternatively, a student could direct the class by performing the desired hand or arm motions or pointing to the chosen words on the board.

Blue sky

Through text and illustrations, the book *Blue sky* (Wood, 2012) shows what the sky looks like in various types of weather (e.g., blue sky, cloud sky, storm sky, rainbow sky). By adding instruments, students experiment with what the sky might sound like in various types of weather. Below are suggested steps to help students create sounds to accompany this book.

- Students sit in a semi-circle with an assortment of percussion instruments placed in the center of the circle.
- The teacher reads the first entry: "Blue Sky".
- The teacher asks the students: "What does a blue sky sound like?"
- A student chooses an instrument.
- The teacher reads the first entry: "Blue Sky" again, after which the student plays the instrument.
- The teacher reads the next entry: "Cloud Sky".
- The teacher asks the students: "What does a cloud sky sound like?"
- A second student chooses an instrument.
- The teacher reads the text of the second entry: "Cloud Sky" again, after which the student plays the instrument.
- The teacher reads from the beginning of the book, "Blue Sky", and the first student plays an instrument. The teacher follows this with "Cloud Sky" and the second student plays an instrument.

This procedure continues as verses are added one-by-one to create an ensemble presentation with readings from the text and sound effects added with percussion instruments. Teachers are encouraged to adjust the steps as needed to devise procedures that are effective in their classrooms. As well, they are encouraged to adapt this process to books of their own choosing.

Expectations for students vary depending on the capabilities of particular individuals. For some students this activity is a way for them to interact with others, choosing an instrument, waiting for the teacher to read the text before playing their instrument, and waiting their turn as other students play their instruments. If and when students are able to do so, they may provide reasons for their instrument choices. Students who are able to do so may explain their choices verbally. The extent to which these explanations indicate technical aspects of music depends on the verbal proficiency and musical understanding of individual students. For example, a student might choose the wow earth bell to represent the *rainbow sky* (illustration 3) because he likes the sound of the instrument; another student chooses a triangle to represent *cloud sky* (illustration 2) because clouds are high and the sounds of the instrument are high. Non-verbal students may point to words that justify their choices. For example, a student might choose between the words *high* and *low* to describe the sounds chosen to represent the *cloud sky*; a child could choose between the words *loud* and *quiet* to indicate storm sky (illustration 4). Many of these instrument choices are subjective. For example, a variety of instruments could be chosen to represent *dark sky* (illustration 8). Thus, an individual student is free to make a personal choice and justify this response as appropriate for that individual.

Personal stories

In the previous activity, the scripts were the texts from published books. In this activity, the teacher substitutes for the published book a personally created story to which the students add an instrumental accompaniment. Personal stories are devised around subject areas relevant to the students' experiences. For example, if a class is going on a field trip to the fire station, perhaps this trip could form the basis for a story. This activity could prepare students for the trip by showing them what to expect. Following their visit, the story could be retold to reinforce what they learned through this experience. As well, a theme could emerge from a child's (or groups of students') special interests. For example, if a student is interested in horses the teacher might invite the class to create a story about horses in the hopes that this will motivate that student to interact with his or her peers.

Going Out for Recess (see Table 6.4) is a story with suggestions for instrumentation. This narrative was developed around what a group of students may like to do in

TABLE 6.4

Story with Instruments: Going Out for Recess

Narrative	Instrumentation
We are in the classroom. The clock on the wall is ticking.	Tick tock block
The bell rings.	Triangle
The children put on their coats and do up their zippers.	Guiro
They put on their boots.	Drum
They run outside to play.	Several instruments played at the same time (e.g., drum, tambourine, agogo bells, woodblock)
Beatrice, Graham, and Byunghee go up the stairs to the slide.	Wood block
They go down the slide.	Cabasa
They do this again.	Woodblock followed by cabasa
Angela, Sunglim, and Ellen play chase.	Drum and tambourine
Ji-yoon, Cameron, and Henry play on the hanging bars.	Agogo bells
Jackie crunches in the snow.	Sand blocks
The school bell rings.	Triangle
The children run into the school.	Woodblock; claves
They take off their boots.	Drum
They unzip their coats.	Guiro
They go to their seats.	Finger cymbals

their school yard. Readers are encouraged to take this story as a model and change the specific content to correspond to their students. Instruments may be adapted based on available choices, taking into account what sorts of sounds might best create aural images for particular activities. The use of personal stories incorporating songs, movements, props, instruments, personal narratives, and picture books is described in Chapter 7: Musical Narratives.

INSTRUMENTAL CONVERSATIONS

Conversation refers to spoken exchanges between two or more people that rely on the expression of thoughts or ideas.[1] In general, a conversation begins with someone who initiates this exchange (the leader) and another who responds to what the leader has said (the follower). While is it possible for people to talk *at* one another without responding to what others have said, the word *conversation* generally assumes that those involved listen to and reply to the individuals around them. In conversation, individuals do not imitate each other; rather, conversation requires that they provide spontaneous responses or reactions to what was said. Conversations are foundational to human communication and to the development of relationships with others.

Contrary to the spontaneity of conversations, the activities students engage in during formal schooling often require that they imitate their teachers. In music class it is assumed that students sing a repertoire of songs by imitating their teachers' singing voices, perform movement sequences imitating their leaders' movements, or play musical instruments in the traditionally correct manner guided by their instructors' actions. This creates challenging environments for students with ASD, many of whom find it difficult to imitate another's actions (Bhat, Landa, & Galloway, 2011; Rogers, Hepburn, Stackhouse, & Werner, 2003; Smith & Bryson, 2007; Williams, Whiten, & Singh, 2004). In this sense, the word *imitation* imposes boundaries on how teachers and students interact. Teachers are the models for competency in music. Students imitate their teachers' actions in order to gain this competency for themselves.

Although students usually imitate their teachers, it can be helpful to create situations in which teachers imitate their students, or even in which students and teachers converse. Adapted from the spontaneous nature of spoken conversations, instrumental conversations allow the students to become the *leaders* and the teachers (or designates such as instructional assistants) to become the *followers* by imitating the students' actions. This is not a strict imitation. Rather, using musical instruments, the followers listen and respond to the students, sometimes directly imitating the student's actions and sometimes surprising their partners by changing what was created. The use of rhythmic conversations in music education settings is clarified through two educational interventions, one describing instrumental conversations using rhythm sticks and the second with hand drums.

Rhythm sticks

Partners sit across from each other, either on the floor or in chairs. The nature of the partnership depends on the teaching context. A child with ASD could be paired with the teacher, an instructional assistant, or a peer. If paired with an adult, the child takes on the role of the leader; if paired with a peer, the partners may take turns as the leader or the follower.

Participants listen to recorded music (see Tables 6.5, 6.6, 6.7,). This music provides an aural template to signal when the activity begins and ends. It also provides an impetus for the interactions and sets the tempo and dynamics. The child begins by performing an action. This could take many forms: the child could tap the two sticks together or slide one stick across the other; the child could tap the sticks on his or her body or on the floor or could tap the partner's sticks or gently tap the sticks on the partner's body. The partner responds with an action without creating an exact imitation of what the child has done. A suggested starting place is for the partner to begin by imitating the child's actions and then changing the actions. For example, the child taps the sticks together. In response the partner taps his or her own sticks and then taps the child's sticks. These interactions continue with each partner performing an action and pausing to see how the other person reacts. Sometimes they play in unison with partners tapping their sticks together, tapping each other's sticks, or tapping chairs, desks, or the floor (depending on where they are sitting). These interactions become a means of musical communication as each partner builds on what the other has offered (Caldwell, 2006).

This teaching strategy is inspired by Field et al. (2010). In their research they studied how children on the autism spectrum responded to an unfamiliar adult who imitated the children's facial expressions, sounds, and movements. They found that

TABLE 6.5

Instrumental Conversations with Rhythm Sticks: Jazz

Artist	Title	Duration	Album	Label	Catalog number
Guaraldi, V.	Linus and Lucy	3:03	A Boy Named Charlie Brown	Fantasy	FCD-8430-2
Guaraldi, V.	Pebble Beach	2:47	A Boy Named Charlie Brown	Fantasy	FCD-8430-2
Jobim, C. A.	Garota de Ipanema	2:34	The Essential Carlos Antonio Jobim	Verve	836 253-2
Muligan, G.	Line for Lyons	2:30	Gerry Mulligan Quartet Featuring Chet Baker	Fantasy	OJCCD-711-2
Peterson, O.	Moten Swing	2:52	Night Train	Verve	314 521 440-2
Vince Guaraldi Trio	Cast Your Fate to the Wind	3:05	Jazz Impressions of Black Orpheus	Fantasy	FCD-8089-2

TABLE 6.6

Instrumental Conversations with Rhythm Sticks: Western Art Music

Composer	Artist(s)	Title	Duration	Album	Label	Catalog number
Albinoni, T.	The London Virtuoso	Concerto in B flat major, op. 9, no. 11 (Movement 3: Allegro)	3:04	Albinoni Oboe Concerti	Naxos	8.550739
Krebs, J. K.	Andrew Bolotowski, flute; Rebecca Pechefsky, harpsichord	Sonata IV in E minor, Polonaise	1:29	Sonatas for Flute and Harpsichord	Quill Classics	1003
Krebs, J. K.	Andrew Bolotowski, flute; Rebecca Pechefsky, harpsichord	Sonata V in A minor, Polonaise	1:36	Sonatas for Flute and Harpsichord	Quill Classics	1003
Poulenc, F.	Alexandre Tharaud, piano; Olivier Dolse, oboe; Kaurent Lefevre, bassoon	Trio for oboe, bassoon, and piano (Movement 3: Rondo: tres vif)	3:21	Complete Chamber Music Volume 1	Naxos	8.55361F
Vivaldi, A.	Failoni Chamber Orchestra	Concerto in D major, RV 453, Allegro	3:05	Vivaldi Oboe Concerti Vol. 1	Naxos	8.550859
Vivaldi, A.	Failoni Chamber Orchestra	Concerto in C major, RV 452, Allegro	2:12	Vivaldi Oboe Concerti Vol. 1	Naxos	8.550859
Warlock, P.	Winchester Cathedral Choir and Nicholas Kraemer	Capriol Suite: Mattachins (Sword Dance)	1:02	The British Music Collection: Peter Warlock	Decca	000289 470 1992 3

TABLE 6.7

Instrumental Conversations with Rhythm Sticks: Indigenous, Folk, New Age, Movie, and Popular

Artist/ Composer	Title	Duration	Album	Label	Catalog number
Chieftains, The	Dublin	2:32	Film Cuts	RCA Victor	09026-68438-2
Nunez, C.	Galician Carol	3:10	Brotherhood of Stars	RCA Victor	74321-45375-2
Nunez, C.	The Flight of the Earls	2:31	Brotherhood of Stars	RCA Victor	74321-45375-2
Joy, G.	Bretan Dance/ Douce Dame Jolie	2:52	Celtic Secrets	Ancient Echoes	AE104CD
Mancini, H.	Baby Elephant Walk	2:42	The Best Of Henri Mancini	BMG Belgium	PA 762/2
Bee Gees	Jive Talkin'	4:19	One Night Only	Polydor	314 559 220-2

children were more interactive with this unfamiliar adult than they were with their own parents. Adapting this idea to rhythmic conversations, teachers may observe that some students with ASD immediately respond to the adult, noticing that this person is copying their actions. An interactive *conversation* seems to emerge naturally from this response. If a student does not initiate the interaction, the partner becomes the instigator, trying to gain the student's attention by tapping the student's sticks or gently tapping the student on the arm or the leg. When the child reacts, the adult becomes the follower in the hopes that the child will take the lead. Some persistence may be necessary. If the child does not respond and take the lead the first time the activity is introduced, try again in subsequent sessions. The child may just need some more time to discover his or her role in this relationship, especially if social interaction is a new and unfamiliar concept.

Rhythm sticks are a viable instrument choice for this activity for many reasons. First, since they are relatively inexpensive teachers may be able to afford sufficient numbers of instruments so that everyone in the class can engage in this activity. Second, rhythm sticks are of different colors so the sticks held by one individual are easily distinguished from those of the partner. Third, they are sturdy enough to be tapped on chairs or desks without sustaining damage. Readers may wish to experiment with other instruments such as drums, chikitas, or wood blocks, to ascertain which instruments are most effective when implementing this activity in their own classrooms.

Drums

This activity is adapted from instrumental conversations with rhythm sticks. One of the primary differences is that in the rhythm sticks activity the students each had their own instrument. For this activity the partners share a drum. As described here, this activity is not supported by recorded music, although teachers could add recorded music if they wish. As with the previous activity, teachers can experiment with other instruments to determine what works best with their students. For the sake of clarity the following description is written as though the partners are a student and a teacher. A variety of individuals could take on the teacher's role including a parent, an instructional assistant, or a peer.

Partners sit on the floor. One drum is shared between them. The drum is placed on the floor so each player has access to the instrument when it is their turn. The teacher signals the beginning of the instrumental dialogue through body language indicating it is the student's turn to play or with a verbal signal such as "drumming." The student plays the drum. When the student pauses, the partner drums. The teacher may choose to play the same rhythm played by the student or, as with the instrumental conversations with rhythm sticks, by copying parts of the student's rhythm but also creating something new. For example, the student taps the drum three times; the teacher taps the drum four times and then indicates it is the student's turn. This exchange of musical ideas continues until, through his or her behavior, the student indicates that he or she is finished with this activity. The teacher may terminate the interactions by putting the drum away or with a verbal explanation such as "all finished."

If the student views this as a solo activity, the teacher might initiate a musical dialogue by saying "my turn." When the teacher is finished playing the drum he or she might use body language to indicate the student has the opportunity to play again. A verbal direction such as "your turn" might be needed to clarify the intent of the game. Verbal directions may be removed once the student understands how the turn-taking proceeds.

Chapter Summary

Playing musical instruments is an ideal way to provide active learning experiences for students with ASD. Playing the beat with percussion instruments is an extension of the physical movements that students perform naturally in response to music. Non-pitched percussion instruments are categorized by what they are made of, how they are played, and the relative ease with which students with ASD are able to coordinate movements to handle the playing techniques required for successful performance. Drums, rhythm sticks, and jingle bells are recommended for initial experiences. Instruments that create greater challenges for eye-hand coordination may be used as students gain proficiency in playing instruments.

Musical instruments lend themselves to a variety of instructional interventions. Teachers can help students refine their aural acuity by identifying instruments by their timbres. Students can practice interpreting gestures by creating sounds that are quiet, loud, fast, or slow in response to a conductor's directions. When used in conjunction with songs, musical instruments create avenues for helping students to increase their understanding of beat and rhythm.

Instruments enhance the imagery emerging from the specific words in songs and also communicate the imagery in picture books. Finally, instrumental conversations provide possibilities for students with ASD to build relationships when a partner copies the student's actions, sometimes through exact imitation and other times by varying what the student has done. Many of these interventions highlight music as nonverbal communication, providing opportunities for individuals with ASD to make connections with others.

Discussion Questions

1. How do students on the autism spectrum benefit from opportunities to play musical instruments?
2. How does playing instruments engage students through multiple perspectives for learning (aural, psychomotor, tactile, visual).
3. What themes would be appropriate for engaging your students in creating personal stories with instruments?
4. How might you adapt the instrumental activities provided here for students in your community?

Note

1. While written exchanges can also be thought of as conversations, the view of conversations presented here is limited to verbal communication as this implies face-to-face interpersonal interactions.

7

MUSICAL NARRATIVES

Integrating Musical Experiences through Storytelling and Drama

IN THIS CHAPTER, storytelling and drama are used to integrate the music activities described in earlier chapters (e.g., singing, moving, listening, and playing instruments) into holistic musical experiences called *musical narratives*. This chapter begins with an explanation of how children on the autism spectrum benefit from experiences with musical narratives. This is followed by an example of a musical narrative designed for children on the autism spectrum called *Festive Fall*. Two musical narratives, *Summer Rainstorm* and *Snow Story*, are posted on the companion website. ⏵

In educational practice, these narratives are improvisatory. Teachers adapt the stories to suit their students and the available materials. Teachers are encouraged to extend the narratives presented here with their own creative ideas and to use the information provided here as a springboard for developing their own musical narratives with their students.

Background

The story telling and drama that underlies musical narratives as described in this chapter guide students' understanding of play within social environments and provide experiential learning about sequence and storytelling through interactive play.

Through musical narratives students acquire an understanding of how stories are built from sequences of events with individual sections interconnecting to form a whole. For example, the musical narrative *Festive Fall* portrays a sequence of five main events:

1. Dawn
2. Walking Though the Town
3. Raking the Leaves
4. Afternoon Siesta
5. Dusk

Each event connects with the preceding incident to create a story with a beginning, a middle, and an end.

Developing the ability to understand the interconnectedness of narrative events is significant for children on the autism spectrum. Individuals with autism spectrum disorder (ASD) often do not recognize patterns and sequences in their environments (Peter, 2009). They also have difficulties understanding the cause and effect in a chain of events (Fein & Dunn, 2007). These challenges partially explain why children on the autism spectrum have difficulties handling changes to established routines and understanding intentions and consequences for their actions (Peter, 2003). The play experiences of these musical narratives are intended to help students understand the interconnectedness of a series of events and to see patterns and sequences in their daily lives. The theme presented is drawn from activities associated with *fall*. Musical narratives can be developed around numerous aspects of the child's day-to-day activities and/or environments.

Musical narratives provide students with opportunities to work on basic life skills like walking to school or playing on the school grounds. Teachers may develop narratives that help students gain familiarity with class routines and to develop social skills such as the ability to take turns when playing musical instruments. Musical narratives may also help students prepare for changes in their environment. For example, if students are taking a field trip to the park, a musical narrative might help students prepare for this outing.

Musical narratives provide students with opportunities for shared experiences among a group of people in the creation of make-believe events. Through fantasy play students may extend their propensity for creative and flexible thought. Environments for pretend play provide children "a reflective window on their play behaviour: the possibility to explore, review and reflect on the implications of their actions and behaviour and those of others in the make-believe context, and to make connections with the real world" (Peter, 2003, p. 27).

Musical narratives are built on an apprenticeship model in which the teacher and other caregivers demonstrate appropriate behaviors. The teacher shapes the narratives to meet the needs of individual students. General features, with benefits for children on the autism spectrum, are highlighted below (adapted and extended from Peter, 2003):

- Musical narratives portray a logical sequence of events with a clear beginning and ending. For example, the *Festive Fall* story might begin with readings from the books *Let it fall* (Cocca-Leffler, 2010), *Leaf jumpers* (Gerber, 2006), or *Count down to fall* (Hawk, 2009). After listening to portions of a story, the students create their own drama as they mime the actions for strolling through the leaves, gathering the leaves, and packing them into bags in preparation for winter. Afterwards, they pretend to enjoy an afternoon siesta. The teacher produces sounds on an owl whistle to signal the coming of dusk.

- Musical narratives provide opportunities for direct interaction with adults and children in make-believe activities. The framework for the narrative is a plan that guides the teacher and students through their interactions. The students' immediate reactions and behaviors guide the outcomes of the narratives in practice. For example, in *Fall Festival*, interactions while pretending to rake leaves may be extended in response to how students interact with the activity. This portion of the narrative may be curtailed if students do not understand and, consequently, do not interact with this make-believe activity. This does not imply that the activity is eliminated. The teacher may rethink the teaching process and return to the task in subsequent sessions. For example, when I first asked students to rake the leaves, they did not understand what I was asking them to do. The next week I added a picture of a child raking leaves as a visual cue. When approached the second time, students more readily understood and engaged in the activity.

- In musical narratives, children join in the whole-group experience in ways most appropriate to their individual needs. Adults model appropriate behaviors and encourage the children to imitate the leader's actions, to incorporate their own ideas, and to expand upon the drama presented. As children's actions and reactions are reinforced, their levels of interaction are enhanced.

The written description of the story created around *Fall Festival* provides information to help teachers bring these stories to life in their classrooms (see Table 7.1). The duration of this performance, estimated at between 20 and 30 minutes, depends in large part on the storytelling style of the teacher and the interaction of the children.

TABLE 7.1

Fall Festival

Narrative	Materials
Part 1: Dawn	Instruments: bell, frog guiro, drums, cymbals, maracas
The sun rises over the town. We hear frogs in the distance as they wake from their sleep. The children stretch and yawn as they wake up. They wipe their eyes and look out the window. Summer has come to an end. It is fall.	Visuals: sun, leaves in fall colors Picture Books: *Let it fall* (Cocca-Leffler (2010); *Leaf jumpers* (Gerber, 2006), *Count down to fall* (Hawk, 2009)
Part 2: Walking Through the Town	Instruments: cabasa, guiro, maracas, egg shakers, sand blocks
We see the leaves on the trees in their bright fall colors: brown, gold, orange, red, and yellow. As we walk along, we hear the crunch of the leaves under our feet.	
Part 3: Raking the Leaves	Instruments: cabasa, guiro, maracas, egg shakers, sand blocks
After playing in the leaves, we go to work. The leaves must be raked and put into bags before the winter snows. We each have a rake. We rake the leaves into three large piles. Now we work with partners. We get our bags for gathering the leaves. One person holds the bag and the other one gathers leaves in his or her arms and puts them in the bag. We scrunch the bag to pack the leaves tightly. Our bag isn't full so we can add some more leaves. We must cooperate with our partner—working together to finish the job. This is hard work.	
Part 4: Afternoon Siesta	Recording: *Early autumn* (Getz,1991)
The children have finished their work.	
Part 5: Dusk	Instruments: owl whistle, cricket, egg shakers (glow in the dark)
The day ends. An owl hoots. He signals the coming of night.	
Our fall day has come to an end. We have seen the fall colors of the leaves: brown, gold, orange, red, and yellow. We have played, running and jumping as we scrunch the leaves under our feet. We have raked the leaves into piles and put them into bags. It has been a busy day. Darkness has come and it is time for sleep.	Visuals: moon, owl

Selected portions of the narrative may be presented in separate class sessions, especially when students are first introduced to the activities that make up these stories. For example, students may experience the raking leaves activity in previous sessions and then incorporate this activity into the complete narrative of *Fall Festival*. The long-term goal is that children experience these stories as intact wholes.

Students need previous experience with a variety of music activities similar to those described in earlier chapters before weaving these activities into longer narratives. These narratives build upon several behaviors and/or skills that students have acquired through previous interactions:

- Students are able to follow a leader's directions.
- Students are able to regulate their behaviors in situations that require them to take turns.
- Students are familiar with the sounds produced by a variety of non-pitched percussion instruments such as cabasa, egg shakers, finger cymbals, and sand blocks.
- Students have previous experience playing the instruments used in the story.
- Students have sufficient abilities in joint attention that they are able to interact with others when provided with appropriate guidance.

As well, musical narratives provide students opportunities to:

- Hear sound-making devices such as whistles that represent birds or animals within a context that helps students to understand what these sounds mean.
- To expand on the themes presented in familiar picture books.

Musical Narrative: Festive Fall

Festive Fall is comprised of five sections: Dawn, Walking Though the Town, Raking the Leaves, Afternoon Siesta, and Dusk. It is recommended that children have previous experience moving to the beat and its subdivisions before dramatizing this narrative.

PART I: DAWN

The narrative begins with a description of a fall morning (see Figure 7.1).
The teacher uses non-pitched percussion instruments to add a soundscape to the text. A bell represents the sun and a frog guiro represents the frogs. Students may pantomime waking from their sleep, accompanied by appropriate instruments

sounds. For example, swishing sounds on cymbals and drums represent stretching and yawning. Maracas represent wiping eyes. Large illustrations of the sun and fall leaves in various colors are posted on the walls of the classroom. This provides visual cues to help the students understand the story. Adult caregivers may provide models for the students by acting out the story.

PART 2: WALKING THROUGH THE TOWN

The narrative continues:

> We watch a soft wind shake the trees.
>   It lifts the leaves and sets them free.
>   Released, they flutter through the air, drifting downward gracefully. (Gerber, 2006. np.)

The teacher may then extend the narrative from this book by describing activities children might engage in while outside on a sunny fall day (see Table 7.1).

In this section, students may pretend they are walking through the leaves following the directions of the *talking drum* (see Chapter 5: Movement and Music). A variety of instrument sounds could be added to this drama including, but not limited to, cabasas, guiros, egg shakers, maracas, and sand blocks. The leader, or other adults, may play the instruments when this story is first presented to the students. Students take on this task when they become familiar with the story.

After the students are familiar with the story and take on the role of playing instruments, the students could be organized in a variety of ways. For example, the group could be divided in half with one half of the students stepping through the leaves and the other half playing instruments. Alternately, the majority of the class could be moving through the leaves and a small group of students (perhaps three or four) could add the sounds of the instruments. This decision is based on the context and the ways in which the activity could be arranged to best meet the educational outcomes devised for individual students.

PART 3: RAKING THE LEAVES

The leader improvises the following narrative:

> In this secion of the narrative, the teacher improvises a story around activities people engage in when raking leaves (see Table 7.1) while the students act out the story.

The teacher draws the narrative out in response to the students' actions or moves the story forward by inserting text when students need an impetus to move their actions forward. Adult caregivers provide models for these actions. As described in the previous section of this narrative, this dramatization could be accompanied by non-pitched percussion instruments.

PART 4: AFTERNOON SIESTA

In this section the teacher improvises a text to describe an afternoon siesta (see Table 7.1). This section is a quiet transition in which students use scarves as a medium for interaction with an instructional assistant while listening to music (see Chapter 4: Listening). Music is chosen around a fall theme. Children who are comfortable with this technique may respond positively to *Early autumn* (Getz, 1991).

PART 5: DUSK

The teacher improvises a narrative to describe the end of the day (see Table 7,1). If possible, reduce the light in the room. The owl whistle represents the hoots of an owl. Visuals of a moon and an owl help to make this more concrete for the children. A soundscape is created with the owl whistle and cricket representing evening sounds. The story comes to a close with an improvised text that summarizes the day.

Chapter Summary

Musical narratives provide students with ASD opportunities to experience music through storytelling and drama, facilitating interactive play and joint attention with adult caregivers (including the teacher or leader and instructional assistants) and peers. The theme chosen for this interactive story relates to the children's everyday lives, facilitating skills such as raking leaves within a context of make-believe. Students are actively involved in storytelling. They play instruments to create aural accompaniments for the stories. They dramatize the narratives through pantomime. Learning through story, drama, and music is improvisational. Starting with the frameworks presented here, teachers carefully observe the reactions of their students and adjust the educational context to meet their needs.

Readers are reminded that the use of musical narratives such as the one presented here is not an instant pre-packaged approach to instruction. Children need several opportunities for guidance through the narrative, with each retelling offering children renewed prospects for interactions with others. As well, the teacher helps students build the drama by improvising a text in response to the engagement of the students.

Individual students react to and interact with these activities in personal ways. Some students readily interact with the activities presented here. Other students need repeated experiences integrating music, movement (drama), props, and instruments before actively engaging in an improvised story such as the *Festive Fall*. In some children acceptance and interplay with the stories may be minimally noticeable or seemingly non-existent. This range of responses reflects the continued challenge of working with children on the autism spectrum. Teachers must be persistent in creating environments rich with possibilities for human interactions and observing students to see how individuals react to this environment. As with these narratives, teaching approaches are not predetermined in a step-by-step approach. Rather, interactions unfold in the moment as teachers respond to students' actions and reactions to their immediate environment.

Discussion Questions

1. How do students with ASD benefit from educational experiences that combine music with drama and storytelling?
2. What themes lend themselves to the development of musical narratives for students in your community?

Forms to Aid the Development of Student Profiles

1. Student profile (initial assessment)

Student _____ **Age** _____

1. What does this student particularly like?

```
┌─────────────────────────────────────────────────────┐
│                                                       │
│                                                       │
│                                                       │
│                                                       │
│                                                       │
└─────────────────────────────────────────────────────┘
```

2. What does this student particularly dislike?

```
┌─────────────────────────────────────────────────────┐
│                                                       │
│                                                       │
│                                                       │
│                                                       │
│                                                       │
└─────────────────────────────────────────────────────┘
```

3. In what situations does this student engage in joint attention?

4. How does this student respond to language?

5. How does this student use language?

6. What, if any, repetitive motions (e.g., rocking, flapping hands) are typically demonstrated by this student?:

7. In what situations, if any, might this student engage in behaviors that may cause injury to the student and/or to others?

8. Which, if any, of the following elements of music does this student respond to? If possible, provide descriptions or explanations for your responses.

   a. songs and singing: _____ yes _____ no _____ do not know

   b. beat and rhythm: _____ yes _____ no _____ do not know

   c. tempo: _____ yes _____ no _____ do not know

   d. dynamics: _____ yes _____ no _____ do not know

9. Overall, how does this student's interest in music rate?

   _____ high

   _____ medium

   _____ low

   _____ none

   _____ do not know

10. What other information will help the music teacher in interacting with this student or in creating music-based programming for this student?

2. Program Profile (initial assessment)

Background Information
Name of student_____ Age of student _____
Educational Context:
inclusion _____ partial inclusion _____
individual instruction _____
other (please describe):

_____
_____

    1. How might this student benefit from this music program?

    2. What strengths do you possess for working with this student?

    3. What approaches or activities in your music class have been successful when working with students with ASD?

    4. How do you anticipate adapting/modifying music instruction for this student?

5. What particular challenges do you anticipate when working with this student?

6. What assistance do you need in developing and implementing a music program for this student?

3. Program Profile (continuing assessment)

Background Information
Name of student_____ Age of student _____
Educational Context:
inclusion _____ partial inclusion _____
individual instruction _____
other (please describe):

_____

_____

1. How has this student benefited from this music program?

2. From a teacher's perspective, what instructional interventions have been particularly successful?

3. How have you adapted/modified music instruction for this student?

4. What adaptations/modifications are planned for future instruction?

5. What assistance do you need as you continue to develop and implement a music program for this student?

6. What are your plans for working with the student during the next school term (or next school year)?

References

Accordino, R., Comer, R., & Heller, W. B. (2007). Searching for music's potential: A critical examination of research on music therapy with individuals with autism. *Research in Autism Spectrum Disorders, 1,* 101–115.

Abramson, R. M. (1997). *Rhythm games for perception & cognition* (rev. ed.). Miami, FL: Warner Bros.

Adamek, M., & Darrow, A. (2010). *Music in special education* (2nd ed.). Silver Spring, MD: American Music Therapy Association.

Alvin, J. (1991). *Music and the autistic child* (2nd ed.). Oxford, UK: Oxford University.

American Psychiatric Association (2013). *Diagnostic and statistical manual of mental disorders* (5th ed.). Washington, DC: American Psychiatric Association.

Anderson, W. M., & Lawrence, J. E. (2010). *Integrating music into the elementary classroom* (8th ed.). Boston, MA: Schirmer Cengage Learning.

Applebaum, E., Egel, A. L., Koegel, R. L., & Imhoff, B. (1979). Measuring musical abilities of autistic children. *Journal of Autism and Developmental Disorders, 9*(3), 279–285.

Armstrong, T. (1999). Research on music and autism: Implications for music educators. *Update: Applications of Research in Music Education, 18*(1), 15–20.

Baranek, G. T. (2002). Efficacy of sensory and motor interventions for children with autism. *Journal of Autism and Developmental Disorders, 32*(5), 397–422.

Barnwell, Y. (1998). *No mirrors in my nana's house.* San Diego, CA: Harcourt Brace & Company.

Bartok, B. (1931). Hungarian sketches [Bear dance & Evening in the village]. On *Bartok concerto for orchestra* [CD]. Canada: BMG (1994).

Berarducci, J. (nd). *Exploring rhythm instruments: An easy guide to teaching and playing the percussion family.* Vancouver, Canada: Empire Music.

Berger, D. S. (2002). *Music therapy, sensory integration and the autistic child.* London, United Kingdom: Jessica Kingsley.

Bernstorf, E. D., & Welsbacher, B. T. (1996). Helping students in the inclusive classroom. *Music Educators Journal, 82*(5), 21–26.

Beurkens, N. (2007). Little steps—big changes. In S. E. Gutstein, H. R. Gutstein, & C. Baird (Eds.). *The relationship development intervention (RDI) program and education* (pp. 9–51). Houston, TX: Connections Center.

Bhat, A. N., Landa, R. J., & Galloway, J. C. (2011). Current perspectives on motor functioning in infants, children, and adults with autism spectrum disorders. *Physical Therapy, 91*(7), 1116–1129.

Birkenshaw-Fleming, L. (1993). *Music for all: Teaching music to people with special needs.* Toronto, Canada: Gordon V. Thompson.

Borczon, R. M. (2004). *Music therapy: A fieldwork primer.* New Braunfels, TX: Barcelona.

Boswell, B. B. (2005). Rhythm, movement and dance. In J. P. Winnick (Ed.), *Adapted physical education and sport* (4th ed., pp. 415–433). Windsor, Canada: Human Kinetics.

Botti, C. (2001). Streets Ahead. On *Night sessions* [CD]. Santa Monica, CA: Columbia.

Boyer, R., & Rozmajzl, M. (2012). *Music: Fundamentals, methods, and materials for the elementary classroom teacher* (5th ed.). Boston, MA: Pearson.

Brock, M. E., & Carter, E. W. (2013). A systematic review of paraprofessional-delivered educational practices to improve outcomes for students with intellectual and developmental disabilities. *Research & Practice for Persons with Severe Disabilities, 38*(4), 211–221.

Bruscia, K. E. (1987). *Improvisational models of music therapy.* Springfield, IL: Charles C. Thomas.

Bruscia, K. E. (1998). *Defining music therapy* (2nd ed.). Gilsum, NH: Barcelona.

Buschner, C. A. (1994). *Teaching children movement concepts and skills: Becoming a master teacher.* Windsor, Canada: Human Kinetics.

Caldwell, P. (2006). Speaking the other's language: Imitation as a gateway to relationship. *Infant and Child Development, 15,* 275–282.

Campbell, P. S., & Scott-Kassner, C. (2006). *Music in childhood: From preschool through the elementary grades* (3rd ed.). Belmont, CA: Thomson Schirmer.

CAST. (2011). *Universal design for learning (UDL) guidelines: Full-text representation, Version 2.0.* Retrieved from http://www.udlcenter.org/aboutudl/udlguidelines

Causton-Theoharis, J. N., Theoharis, G. T., & Trezek, B. J. (2008). Teaching pre-service teachers to design inclusive instruction: A lesson planning template. *International Journal of Inclusive Education, 12*(4), 381–399.

Centelles, L., Assaiante, C., Etchegoyhen, K., Bouvard, M., & Schmitz, C. (2013). From action to interaction: Exploring the contribution of body motion cues to social understanding in typical development and in autism spectrum disorders. *Journal of Autism and Developmental Disorders, 43,* 1140–1150.

Choksy, L. (1999). *The Kodaly method I: Comprehensive music education* (3rd ed.). Upper Saddle River, NJ: Prentice-Hall.

Choksy, L., Abramson, R. M., Gillespie, A. E., Woods, D., & York, F. (2001). *Teaching music in the twenty-first century* (2nd ed.). Upper Saddle River, NJ: Prentice Hall.

Cocca-Leffler, M. (2010). *Let it fall.* New York, NY: Scholastic.

Corke, M. (2002). *Approaches to communication through music.* London, United Kingdom: David Fulton.

Darrow, A. A. (2007). Adaptations in the classroom: Accommodations and modifications (Part 1). *General Music Today, 20*(3), 32–34.

Darrow, A. A. (2008). Adaptations in the classroom: Accommodations and modifications (Part II). *General Music Today, 21*(3), 32–34.

Darrow, A. A. (2009). Adapting for students with autism. *General Music Today, 22*(2), 24–26.

Darrow, A. A. (2010). Music education for all: Employing the principles of Universal Design to educational practice. *General Music Today, 24*(1), 43–45.

Dean, J. (2013). *Pete the cat: The wheels on the bus.* New York, NY: Harper.

Dean, J. (2014). *Pete the cat: Twinkle, twinkle, little star.* New York, NY: Harper.

Dempsey, I., & Forman, P. (2001). A review of educational approaches for individuals with autism. *International Journal of Disability, Development, and Education, 48*(1), 103–116.

Dimitriadis, T., & Smeijsters, H. (2011). Autistic spectrum disorder and music therapy: Theory undermining practice. *Nordic Journal of Music Therapy, 20*(2), 108–122.

Donnell, N. E. (2007). Messages through the music: Musical dialogue as a means of communicative dialogue. *Canadian Journal of Music Therapy, 13*(2), 74–102.

Dowd, A. M., McGinley, J. L., Taffe, J. R., & Rinehart, N. J. (2012). Do planning and visual integration difficulties underpin motor dysfunction in autism? A kinematic study of young children with autism. *Journal of Autism and Developmental Disorders, 42*(8), 1539–1548.

Dylan, B., & Muth, J. J. (2011). *Blowin' in the wind.* New York, NY: Sterling Children's Books.

Dziuk, M. A., Gidley-Larson, J. C., Apostu, A., Mshone, E. M., Denkla, M. B., & Mostofsky, S. H. (2007). Dyspraxia in autism: Association with motor, social, and communicative deficits. *Developmental Medicine & Child Neurology, 49,* 734–739.

Earl, L. (2003). *Assessment as learning: Using classroom assessment to maximize student learning.* Thousand Oaks, CA: Corwin.

Engel, C. & Songs, S. (2008). *Knick knack paddy whack.* Cambridge, MA: Barefoot books.

Evans, C., Williams, J. B., King, L., & Metcalf, D. (2010). Modeling, guided instruction, and application of UDL in a rural special education teacher preparation program. *Rural Special Education Quarterly, 29*(4), 41–48.

Fatus, S., & Penner, F. (2007). *Here we go round the mulberry bush.* Cambridge, MA: Barefoot books.

Feierabend, J. M., & Kahan, J. (2003). *The book of movement exploration: Can you move like this?* Chicago, IL: GIA.

Fein, D., & Dunn, M. (2007). *Autism in your classroom: A general educator's guide to students with autism spectrum disorder.* Bethesda, MD: Woodbine House.

Field, T., Nadel, J., Diego, M., Hernndez-Reif, M., Russo, K., Vchulek, D., Lendi, K., & Siddalingappa, V. (2010). Children with autism are more imitative with an imitative adult than with their parents. *Early Development and Care, 180*(4), 513–518.

Frazee, M. (1999). *Hush little baby.* New York, NY: Harcourt.

Frith, U. (1972). Cognitive mechanisms in autism: Experiments with color and tone sequence production. *Journal of Autism and Clinical Childhood Schizophrenia, 2*(2), 160–173.

Gardstrom, S. C. (2007). *Music therapy improvisation for groups: Essential leadership competencies.* Gilsum, NH: Barcelona.

Gerber, C. (2006). *Leaf jumpers.* Watertown, MA: Charlesbridge.

Getz, S. (1991). *The artistry of Stan Getz: The best of the Verve years, volume 1*[CD] New York, NY: Verve D225113.

Gluck, C. W. (1762). Dance of the blessed spirits [Recorded by Nora Shulman and Judy Loman]. On *Dance of the blessed spirits* [CD]. Hong Kong: Naxos. (1997)

Gooding, L. (2009). Enhancing social competence in the music classroom. *General Music Today*, *23*(1), 35–38.

Hackett, P., & Lindeman, C. A. (2004). *The musical classroom: Backgrounds, models, and skills for elementary teaching* (6th ed.). Upper Saddle River, NJ: Pearson.

Hallett, M., Lebiedowska, M. K., Thomas, S. L., Stanhope, S. J., Denckla, M. B., & Runsey, J. (1993). Locomotion of autistic adults. *Archives of Neurology*, *50*(12), 1304–1308.

Hammel, A. M., & Hourigan, R. M., (2011). *Teaching music to students with special needs: A label-free approach*. New York, NY: Oxford.

Hammel, A. M., & Hourigan, R. M. (2013). *Teaching music to students with autism*. New York, NY: Oxford.

Hardy, M. W., & LaGasse, A. B. (2013). Rhythm, movement, and autism: Using rhythmic rehabilitation research as a model for autism. *Frontiers in Integrative Neuroscience*, *7*, 1–9.

Harter, D. (2000). *The animal boogie*. Cambridge, MA: Barefoot books.

Hawk, F. (2009). *Count down to fall*. Mt. Pleasant, NC: Sylvan Dell.

Heaton, P. (2003). Pitch memory, labelling, and disembedding in autism. *Journal of Psychology and Psychiatry*, *44*(4), 543–551.

Heaton, P. (2005). Interval and contour processing in autism. *Journal of Autism and Developmental Disorders*, *35*(6), 787–793.

Heaton, P., Hermelin, B., & Pring, L. (1998). Autism and pitch processing: A precursor for savant musical ability? *Music Perception*, *15*(3), 291–305.

Heaton, P., Pring, L., & Hermelin, B. (1999). A pseudo-savant: A case of exceptional musical splinter skills. *Neurocase*, *5*, 503–509.

Hedden, D. (2012). An overview of existing research about children's singing and the implications for teaching children to sing. *Update: Applications of Research in Music Education*, *30*(2), 52–62.

Herrold, R. M. (2001). *New approaches to elementary classroom music* (3rd ed.). Upper Saddle River, NJ: Prentice Hall.

Heutig, C., Pyfer, J., & Auxter, D. (2001). *Gross motor activities for young children with special needs* (9th ed.). Toronto, Canada: McGraw-Hill.

Hilton, C. L., Zhang, Y., White, M. R., Klohr, C. L., & Constantine, J. (2011). Motor impairment in sibling pairs concordant and discordant for autism spectrum disorders. *Autism*, *16*(4), 430–441.

Hobson, P. R., & Lee, A. (1999). Imitation and identification in autism. *Journal of Child Psychology & Psychiatry*, *40*(4), 649–659.

Hort, L. (2000). *The seals on the bus*. New York, NY: Henry Holt.

Hughes, C. (1996). Brief report: Planning problems in autism at the level of motor control. *Journal of Autism and Developmental Disorders*, *26*(1), 99–107.

Ingersoll, B., & Schreibman, L. (2006). Teaching reciprocal imitation skills to young children with autism. *Journal of Autism and Developmental Disorders*, *36*(4), 487–505.

Innocenti, A., De Stefani, E., Bernardi, N. F., Campione, G. C., & Gentilucci, M. (2012). Gaze direction and request gesture in social interactions. *Public Library of Science*, *7*(5), 1–8.

Iseminger, S. H. (2009). Keys to success with autistic children: Structure, predictability, and consistency are essential for students on the autism spectrum. *Teaching Music*, *16*(6), 28–31.

Johnson, F. (2002). Models of service delivery and their relation to the IEP. In B. L. Wilson, (Ed.), *Models of music therapy in school settings* (pp. 83–107). Silver Spring, MD: American Music Therapy Association.

Jones, E. A., & Carr, E. G. (2004). Joint attention in children with autism: Theory and intervention. *Focus on Autism and Other Developmental Disabilities, 19*(1), 13–26.

Katz, J. (2012). *Teaching to diversity: The three-block model of Universal Design for Learning.* Winnipeg, Canada: Portage & Main.

Kern, P., Graham, F. P., Aldridge, D. (2006). Using embedded music therapy interventions to support outdoor play of young children with autism in an inclusive community-based child care program. *Journal of Music Therapy, 43*(4), 270–294.

Kern, P., Wolery, M., & Aldridge, D. (2007). Use of songs to promote independence in morning greeting routines for young children with autism. *Journal of Autism and Developmental Disorders, 37,* 1264–1271.

Kim, J. (2000). Children's pitch matching, vocal range, and developmentally appropriate practice. *Journal of Research in Childhood Education, 14*(2), 152–160.

Kovalski, M. (1987). *The wheels on the bus.* Toronto, Canada: Kids Can.

Kranowitz, C. S. (2006a). *The out-of-sync child has fun: Activities for kids with sensory processing disorder.* New York, NY: Perigee.

Kranowitz, C. S. (2006b). *The out-of-sync child: Recognizing and coping with sensory processing disorder.* New York, NY: Perigee.

Krikeli, V., Michailidis, A., & Klavdianou, N. D. (2010). Communication improvement through music: The case of children with developmental disabilities. *International Journal of Special Education, 25*(1), 1–9.

Lagasse, A. B., & Hardy, M. W. (2013). Considering rhythm for sensorimotor regulation in children with autism spectrum disorders. *Music Therapy Perspectives, 31,* 67–77.

Landy, J. M., & Burridge, K. R. (1999). *Ready-to-use fundamental motor skills and movement activities for young children: Teaching, assessment & remediation.* West Nyack, NY: The Center for Applied Research in Education.

Lawson, J. (2003). Depth accessibility difficulties: An alternative conceptualization of autism spectrum conditions. *Journal for the Theory of Social Behavior, 33*(2), 189–202.

Lightfoot, G., & Wallace, I. (2010). *Canadian railroad trilogy.* Toronto, Canada: Groundwood Books/House of Anansi.

Lim, H. A. (2012). *Developmental speech-language training through music for children with autism spectrum disorders: Theory and clinical application.* London, United Kingdom: Jessica Kingsley.

Lytle, R., & Todd, T. (2009). Stress and the student with autism spectrum disorders: Strategies for stress reduction and enhanced learning. *Teaching Exceptional Children, 41*(4), 36–42.

Mace, R. L., Story, M. F., & Mueller, J. L. (1998). A brief history of universal design. In *The universal design file: Designing for people of all ages and abilities* (pp. 5–14). Raleigh, NC: Center for Universal Design, North Caroline State University.

Maljaars, M., Noens, I., Jansen, R., Scholte, E., & van Berckelaer-Onnes, I. (2011). Intentional communication in nonverbal and verbal low-functioning children with autism. *Journal of Communication Disorders, 44,* 601–614.

Mancini, H. (1997). *Baby elephant walk.* On *The Best of Henri Mancini.* Belgium: BMG.

Manitoba Education and Youth. (2003). *Independent together: Supporting the multilevel learning community.* Winnipeg, Canada: The Crown in Right of Manitoba.

Manning, M. M., & Wainwright, L. D. (2010). The role of high level play as a predictor of social functioning in autism. *Journal of Autism and Developmental Disorders, 40*, 523–533.

Mari, M., Castiello, U., Marks, D., Marraffa, C., & Prior, M. (2003). The reach-to-grasp movement in children with autism spectrum disorder. *Philosophical Transactions of the Royal Society, 358*(1430), 393–403.

McGuire, J. M., Scott, S. S., & Shaw, S. F. (2006). Universal design and its applications in educational environments. *Remedial and Special Education, 27*(3), 166–175.

McMillan, E., & Saffran, J. R. (2004). Music and language: A developmental comparison. *Music Perception, 21*(3), 289–311.

McQuinn, A., & Fatus, S. (2009). *If you're happy and you know it.* Cambridge, MA: Barefoot Books.

Montgomery, A. P. (2002). *Teaching towards musical understanding: A handbook for the elementary grades.* Toronto, Canada: Pearson Education Canada.

Morin, B., & Reid, G. (1985). A quantitative and qualitative assessment of autistic individuals on selected motor tasks. *Adapted Physical Activity Quarterly, 2*, 43–55.

Nind, M. (2000). Intensive interaction and children with autism. In S. Powell (Ed.), *Helping children with autism to learn* (pp. 39–49). London, United Kingdom: David Fulton.

No author. (2008). *Old MacDonald had a farm (a pop-up book).* Sywel, United Kingdom: Igloo.

Nordoff, P., & Robbins, C. (2007). *Creative music therapy: A guide to fostering clinical musicianship* (2nd ed.). Gilsum, NH: Barcelona.

Nordoff, P., & Robbins, C. (1971). *Music therapy in special education.* New York, NY: J. Day.

Notbohm, E. (2006). *Ten things your student with autism wishes you knew.* Arlington, TX: Living Horizons.

Obiakor, F. E., Harris, M., Mutua, K., Rotatori, A., & Algozzine, B. (2012). Making inclusion work in general education classrooms. *Education and Treatment of Children, 35*(3), 477–490.

O'Brien, J. (2000). *The farmer in the dell.* Honesdale. PA: Boyds Mills.

Ockelford, A. (2000). Music in education of children with severe or profound learning difficulties: Issues in current UK provision, a new conceptual framework, and proposals for research. *Psychology of Music, 28*, 197–217.

Paparella, T., Goods, K. S., Freeman, S., & Kasari, C. (2011). The emergence of nonverbal joint attention and requesting skills in young children with autism. *Journal of Communication Disorders, 44*, 569–583.

Peter, M. (2003). Drama, narrative, and early learning. *British Journal of Special Education, 30*(1), 21–27.

Peter, M. (2009). Drama: Narrative pedagogy and socially challenged children. *British Journal of Special Education, 36*(1), 9–17.

Preston, D., & Carter, M. (2009). A review of the efficacy of the picture exchange communication system intervention. *Journal of Autism and Developmental Disorders, 39*(11), 1471–1486.

Prizant, B. M. (1983). Language acquisition and communicative behavior in autism: Toward an understanding of the "whole" of it. *Journal of Speech and Hearing Disorders, 48*, 296–307.

Prizant, B. M. (1987). Theoretical and clinical implications of echolalic behavior in autism. In T. Layton (Ed.), *Language and treatment of autistic and developmentally disordered children* (pp. 65–88). Springfield, IL: Charles C. Thomas.

Prizant, B. M., & Duchan, J. F. (1981). The functions of immediate echolalia in autistic children. *Journal of Speech and Hearing Disorders, 46*, 241–249.

Prizant, B. M., Schuler, A. L., Wetherby, A. M., & Rydell, P. (1997). Enhancing language and communication development: Language approaches. In D. Cohen & F. Volkmar (Eds.), *Handbook of autism and pervasive developmental disorders* (pp. 572–605). Hoboken, NJ: Wiley.

Raposo, J., & Lichtenheld, T. (2013). *Sing.* New York, NY: Henry Holt.

Reed, S. & Oldfield, R. (2010). *Up, up, up.* Cambridge, MA: Barefoot books.

Rinehart, N. J., Bradshaw, J. L., Brereton, A. V., & Tonge, B. J. (2001). Movement preparation in high-functioning autism and Asperger disorder: A serial choice reaction time task involving motor reprogramming. *Journal of Autism and Developmental Disorders, 31*(1), 79–88.

Roberts, S., & Bell, S. (2003). *We all go traveling by.* Cambridge, MA: Barefoot Books.

Rodgers, R., & Hammerstein, O. (2001). *My favorite things.* New York, NY: HarperTrophy.

Rodgers, J., Glod, M., Connolly, B., & McConachie, H. (2012). The relationship between anxiety and repetitive behaviours in autism spectrum disorder. *Journal of Autism and Developmental Disorders, 42*, 2404–2409.

Rogers, S. J., Bennetto, L., McEvoy, R., & Pennington, B. F. (1996). Imitation and pantomime in high-functioning adolescents with autism spectrum disorders. *Child Development, 67*, 2060–2073.

Rogers, S. J., Hepburn, S. L., Stackhouse, T., & Werner, E. (2003). Imitation performance in toddlers with autism and those with other developmental disorders. *Journal of Child Psychology and Psychiatry, 44*(5), 763–781.

Rose, D. L., & Armstrong-Ellis, C. (2009). *The twelve days of springtime: A school counting book.* New York, NY: Abrams books for young readers.

Rutherford, M. D., Young, G. S., Hepburn, S., & Rogers, S. J. (2007). A longitudinal study of pretend play in autism. *Journal of Autism and Developmental Disorders, 37*, 1024–1039.

Rydell, P. J., & Prizant, B. M. (1995). Assessment and intervention strategies for children who use echolalia. In K. Quill (Ed.), *Teaching children with autism* (pp. 105–129). New York, NY: Delmar.

Saint-Saëns, C. (1886). The carnival of the animals. On *The carnival of the animals; Peter and the wolf; The young person's guide to the orchestra* [CD]. Hong Kong: Naxos. (1990)

Sausser, S. (2006). A model for music therapy with students with emotional and behavioral disorders. *The Arts in Psychotherapy, 33*, 1–10.

Schmitz, C., Martineau, J., Barthélémy, C., & Assaiante, C. (2003). Motor control and children with autism: Deficit of anticipatory function? *Neuroscience Letters, 348*(1), 17–20.

Schon, D., Boyer, M., Moreno, S., Besson, M., Peretz, I., & Kolinsky, R. (2008). Songs as an aid for language acquisition. *Cognition 106*(2), 975–983.

Schreibman, L., & Carr, E. G. (1978). Elimination of echolalic responding to questions through the training of a generalized verbal response. *Journal of Applied Behavior Analysis, 11*(4), 453–463.

Scott, S. J. (2012). Rethinking the roles of assessment in music education. *Music Educators Journal, 98*(3), 31–35

Scott, S. J. (2016). The challenges of imitation for children with autism spectrum disorders with implications for general music education. *Update: Applications of research in Music Education, 34*(2), 13–20.

Secret Garden (1995). *Songs from a secret garden* [CD]. Santa Monica, CA: Universal Music.

Shore, S. M. (2003). The language of music: Working with children on the autistic spectrum. *Journal of Education, 183*(2), 97–108.

Shulman, L. (2002). *Old MacDonald had a woodshop*. New York, NY: G. P. Putnam.

Simpson, K., & Keen, D. (2011). Music interventions for children with autism: Narrative review of the literature. *Journal of Autism and Developmental Disorders, 41*(11), 1507–1514.

Simpson, K., Keen, D., & Lamb, J. (2013). The use of music to engage children with autism in a receptive labelling task. *Research in Autism Spectrum Disorders, 7*, (2013). 1489–1496.

Sinclaire, D. (2003). Still got it. On *Denzal Sinclaire* [CD]. Toronto, Canada: Verve. CD-4400385782

Sinclaire, D. (2003). Tofu and greens. On *Denzal Sinclaire* [CD]. Toronto, Canada: Verve. CD-4400385782

Slavin, B. (1992). *The cat came back*. Toronto, Canada: Kids Can Press.

Smith, I. M., & Bryson, S. E. (2007). Gesture imitation in autism: II. Symbolic gestures and pantomimed object use. *Cognitive Neuropsychology, 24*(7), 679–700.

Spiker, M. A., Lin, C. E., Van Dyke, M., & Wood, J. J. (2012). Restricted interests and anxiety in children with autism. *Autism, 16*(3), 306–320.

Staples, K. L., & Reid, G. (2010). Fundamental movement skills and autism spectrum disorders. *Journal of Autism and Developmental Disorders, 40*(2), 209–217.

Starr, R., & Cort, B. (2014). *Octopus's garden*. New York, NY: Aladdin.

Steen, A. (1992). *Exploring Orff: A teacher's guide*. Mainz, NY: Schott.

Stott, D. (2010). *Ten in the bed*. Stow, OH: Twin Sisters.

Streeter, E. (1993). *Making music with the young child with special needs: A guide for parents* (Rev. ed.). London, United Kingdom: Jessica Kingsley.

Sumway-Cook, A., & Woollacott, M. H. (2007). *Motor control: Translating research into clinical practice* (3rd ed.). Philadelphia, PA: Lippincott Williams & Wilkins.

Szatmari, P., Bryson S. E., Boyle, M. H., Streiner, D. L., & Duku, E. (2003). Predictors of outcome among high functioning children with autism and Asperger syndrome. *Journal of Child Psychology and Psychiatry and Allied Disciplines, 44*(4), 520–528.

Taylor, C., & Stephens, P. (2002). *Out on the prairie: A Canadian counting book*. Toronto, Canada: Scholastic.

Temple, C., Martinez, M., Yokota, J., & Naylor, A. (2002). *Children's books in children's hands: An introduction to their literature* (2nd ed.). Boson, MA: Allyn and Bacon.

Terpstra, J. E., Higgins, K., & Pierce, T. (2002). Can I play? Classroom-based interventions for teaching play skills to children with autism. *Focus on Autism & Other Developmental Disabilities, 17*(2), 119–126.

Thaut, M. (1987). Visual versus auditory (musical) stimulus preferences in autistic children: A pilot study. *Journal of Autism and Developmental Disorders, 17*, 425–432.

Thaut, M. H. (2008). *Rhythm, music, and the brain*. New York, NY: Routledge.

Todd, T. (2012). Teaching motor skills to individuals with autism spectrum disorders. *Journal of Physical Education, Recreation & Dance, 83*(8), 32–48.

Trapani, I. (2004). *How much is that doggie in the window?* Watertown, MA: Charlesbridge.

Travis, L., Sigman, M., & Ruskin, E. (2001). Links between social understanding and social behavior in verbally able children with autism. *Journal of Autism and Developmental Disorders, 31*(2), 119–130.

Trollinger, V. (2007). Pediatric vocal development and voice science: Implications for teaching singing. *General Music Today, 20*(3), 19–25.

Underwood, D., & Liwska, R. (2010). *The quiet book*. Boston, MA: Houghton Mifflin Books for Children.

Underwood, D., & Liwska, R. (2011). *The loud book*. Boston, MA: Houghton Mifflin Books for Children.

Vaiouli, P., Grimmet, K., & Ruich, L. J., (2015). "Bill is now singing": Joint engagement and the emergence of social communication of three young children with autism. *Autism, 19*(1), 73–83.

Vanvuchelen, M., Roeyers, H., & De Weerdt, W. (2007). Nature of motor imitation problems in school-aged boys with autism: A motor or a cognitive problem? *Autism, 11*(3), 225–240.

Vernazza-Martin, S., Martin, N., Vernazza, A., Lepellec-Muller, A., Rufo, M., Massion, J. (2005). Goal directed locomotion and balance control in autistic children. *Journal of Autism and Developmental Disorders, 35*(1), 91–102.

Vetter, J. R. (2009). *Down by the station*. Berkeley, CA: Tricycle Press.

Vivanti, G., Nadig, A., Ozonoff, S., & Rogers, S. J. (2008). What do children with autism attend to during imitation tasks? *Journal of Experimental Psychology, 101*, 186–205.

Wadsworth, O.A., & Vojtech, A. (2002). *Over in the meadow*. New York, NY: North-South.

Wan, C. Y., Demaine, K., Zipse, L., Norton, A., & Schlang, G. (2010). From music making to speaking: Engaging the mirror neuron system in autism. *Brain Research Bulletin, 82*, 161–168.

Warlock, P. (1926). Capriol suite (pied-en l'air) [Recorded by Academy of St Martin in the Fields]. On *The British music collection: Peter Warlock-capriol suite, serenade for strings, lullaby my Jesus* [CD]. London, UK: Decca. (2004)

Watson, L. R., Roberts, J. E., Baranek, G. T., Mandulak, K. C., & Dalton, J. C. (2012). Behavioral and physiological responses to child-directed speech of children with autism spectrum disorders of typical development. *Journal of Autism and Developmental Disorders, 42*(8), 1616–1629.

Weidner, T. (2009). *Sleep, baby, sleep*. Wilton, CT: Tiger Tales.

Wigham, S., Rodgers, S., South, M., McConachie, H., & Freeston, M. (2015). The interplay between sensory processing abnormalities, intolerance of uncertainty, anxiety and restricted and repetitive behaviours in autism spectrum disorder. *Journal of Autism and Developmental Disorders, 45*, 943–952.

Williams, J. H. G., Whiten, A., & Singh, T. (2004). A systematic review of action imitation in autistic spectrum disorders. *Journal of Autism and Developmental Disorders, 34*(3), 285–299.

Wood, A. (2012). *Blue sky*. New York, NY: Blue sky press.

Wood. D. (1996). *Move, sing, listen, play* (Rev. ed.). Toronto, Canada: Gordon V. Thompson.

Yang, T., Wolfberg, P. J., Wu, S., & Hwu, P. (2003). Supporting children on the autism spectrum in peer play at home and school. *Autism: The International Journal of Research and Practice, 7*(4), 437–453.

Yarrow, P., & Lipton, L. (2007). *Puff, the magic dragon*. New York, NY: Sterling.

Yarrow, P., & Sweet, M. (2009). *Day is done*. New York, NY: Sterling.

Zhang, J., & Griffin, A. J. (2007). Including children with autism in general physical education: Eight possible solutions. *The Journal of Physical Education, Recreation & Dance, 28*(3), 33–50.

Bibliography of Suggested Resources

Adamek, M., & Darrow, A. (2010). *Music in special education* (2nd ed.). Silver Spring, MD: American Music Therapy Association.

Darrow, A. A. (2007). Adaptations in the classroom: Accommodations and modifications (Part 1). *General Music Today, 20*(3), 32–34.

Darrow, A. A. (2008). Adaptations in the classroom: Accommodations and modifications (Part 2). *General Music Today, 21*(3), 32–34.

Darrow, A. A. (2009). Adapting for students with autism. *General Music Today, 22*(2), 24–26.

Darrow, A. A. (2010). Music education for all: Employing the principles of Universal Design to educational practice. *General Music Today, 24*(1), 43–45.

Fein, D., & Dunn, M. (2007). *Autism in your classroom: A general educator's guide to students with autism spectrum disorder.* Bethusda, MD: Woodbine House.

Hammel, A. M., & Hourigan, R. M., (2011). *Teaching music to students with special needs: A label-free approach.* New York, NY: Oxford.

Hammel, A. M., & Hourigan, R. M. (2013). *Teaching music to students with autism.* New York, NY: Oxford.

Kranowitz, C. S. (2006). *The out-of-sync child has fun: Activities for kids with sensory processing disorder.* New York, NY: Perigee.

Kranowitz, C. S. (2006). *The out-of-sync child: Recognizing and coping with sensory processing disorder.* New York, NY: Perigee.

Lim, H. A. (2012). *Developmental speech-language training through music for children with autism spectrum disorders: Theory and clinical application.* London, United Kingdom: Jessica Kingsley.

Scott, S. J. (2016). The challenges of imitation for children with autism spectrum disorders with implications for general music education. *Update: Applications of research in Music Education, 34*(2), 13–20.

Wood. D. (1996). *Move, sing, listen, play* (rev. ed.). Toronto, Canada: Gordon V. Thompson.

Index